Clinical Examinati
in Paediatrics

T0176769

Clinical Examination Skills in Paediatrics

For MRCPCH Candidates and Other Practitioners

Edited by

A. Mark Dalzell
Retired Consultant Paediatric Gastroenterologist
Alder Hey Children's NHS Foundation Trust
Liverpool
UK

Ian Sinha
Consultant in Paediatric Respiratory Medicine
Honorary Senior Lecturer in Child Health
Alder Hey Children's NHS Foundation Trust
Liverpool
UK

WILEY Blackwell

Registered Office(s)
John Wiley & Sons, Inc., 111 River Street, Hoboken, NJ 07030, USA
John Wiley & Sons Ltd, The Atrium, Southern Gate, Chichester, West Sussex, PO19 8SQ, UK

Editorial Office
9600 Garsington Road, Oxford, OX4 2DQ, UK

For details of our global editorial offices, customer services, and more information about Wiley products visit us at www.wiley.com.

Wiley also publishes its books in a variety of electronic formats and by print-on-demand. Some content that appears in standard print versions of this book may not be available in other formats.

Library of Congress Cataloging-in-Publication Data
Names: Dalzell, A. Mark, editor. | Sinha, Ian, editor.
Title: Clinical examination skills in paediatrics : for MRCPCH candidates and other practitioners / [edited by] Mark Dalzell, Ian Sinha.
Description: Hoboken, NJ : Wiley-Blackwell, 2020. | Includes bibliographical references and index.
Identifiers: LCCN 2019035290 (print) | LCCN 2019035291 (ebook) | ISBN 9781118746080 (paperback) | ISBN 9781119238850 (adobe pdf) | ISBN 9781119238935 (epub)
Subjects: MESH: Diagnostic Techniques and Procedures | Child
Classification: LCC RJ50 (print) | LCC RJ50 (ebook) | NLM WS 141 | DDC 618.92/0075–dc23
LC record available at https://lccn.loc.gov/2019035290
LC ebook record available at https://lccn.loc.gov/2019035291

Cover Design: Wiley
Cover Images: Little boy crouching and Father with his baby © Westend61/Getty Images, Affectionate mother © Hoxton/Sam Edwards/Getty Images, Girl playing toy cars © 10'000 Hours/Getty Images

Set in 11/13.5pt Minion Pro by SPi Global, Pondicherry, India
Printed and bound in Singapore by Markono Print Media Pte Ltd

10 9 8 7 6 5 4 3 2 1

Contents

List of contributors

Editors

A. Mark Dalzell
Retired Consultant Paediatric Gastroenterologist
Alder Hey Children's NHS Foundation Trust
Liverpool
UK

Ian Sinha
Consultant in Paediatric Respiratory Medicine
Honorary Senior Lecturer in Child Health
Alder Hey Children's NHS Foundation Trust
Liverpool
UK

Chapter authors

Richard E. Appleton
Department of Paediatric Neurology
The Roald Dahl Neurophysiology Department
Alder Hey Children's NHS Foundation Trust
Liverpool
UK

Michael T. Bowes
Department of Paediatric Cardiology
Alder Hey Children's NHS Foundation Trust
Liverpool
UK

Gavin Cleary
Department of Paediatric Rheumatology
Alder Hey Children's NHS Foundation Trust
Liverpool
UK

Urmi Das
Department of Paediatric Endocrinology
Alder Hey Children's NHS Foundation Trust
Liverpool
UK

Mark Deakin
Department of Paediatric Diabetes
Alder Hey Children's NHS Foundation Trust
Liverpool
UK

Poonam Dharmaraj
Department of Paediatric Endocrinology
Alder Hey Children's NHS Foundation Trust
Liverpool
UK

Ruairi Gallagher
Department of Developmental Paediatrics
Alder Hey Children's NHS Foundation Trust
Liverpool
UK

Melissa Gladstone
Department of Women and Children's Health
Institute of Translational Medicine
University of Liverpool
Alder Hey Children's NHS Foundation Trust
Liverpool
UK

Clare P. Halfhide
Department of Paediatric Respiratory Medicine
Alder Hey Children's NHS Foundation Trust
Liverpool
UK

Daniel B. Hawcutt
Department of Women and Children's Health
Institute of Translational Medicine
University of Liverpool
Alder Hey Children's NHS Foundation Trust
Liverpool
UK

Anand S. Iyer
Department of Paediatric Neurology
Alder Hey Children's NHS Foundation Trust
Liverpool
UK

Caroline B. Jones
Department of Paediatric Cardiology
Alder Hey Children's NHS Foundation Trust
Liverpool
UK

Rachel Kneen
Department of Paediatric Neurology
Alder Hey Children's NHS Foundation Trust
Liverpool
UK

Anastasia Konidari
Department of Paediatric Gastroenterology
Alder Hey Children's NHS Foundation Trust
Liverpool
UK

Sarah J. Mayell
Department of Paediatric Respiratory Medicine
Alder Hey Children's NHS Foundation Trust
Liverpool
UK

Antonia K.S. McBride
Department of Paediatric Respiratory Medicine
Alder Hey Children's NHS Foundation Trust
Liverpool
UK

Liza J. McCann
Department of Paediatric Rheumatology
Alder Hey Children's NHS Foundation Trust
Liverpool
UK

Renuka Ramakrishnan
Department of Paediatric Endocrinology
Alder Hey Children's NHS Foundation Trust
Liverpool
UK

Andrew Riordan
Department of Paediatric Infectious Diseases and Immunology
Alder Hey Children's NHS Foundation Trust
Liverpool
UK

Anna Shawcross
Department of Paediatric Respiratory Medicine
Royal Manchester Children's Hospital
Manchester
UK

Kevin W. Southern
Department of Women and Children's Health
Institute in the Park
University of Liverpool
Alder Hey Children's NHS Foundation Trust
Liverpool
UK

Stefan Spinty
Department of Paediatric Neurology
Alder Hey Children's NHS Foundation Trust
Liverpool
UK

Dean Wallace
Department of Paediatric Nephrology
Royal Manchester Children's Hospital
Manchester
UK

How to use this book

Ian Sinha and A. Mark Dalzell

This book and the accompanying companion website have been produced to aid MRCPCH students, but we hope that they will be a useful teaching and learning tool for any practitioner of paediatrics.

The opportunity and privilege to work with children and their families, together with colleagues who are committed to providing quality care, is something that one simply cannot put a value on. The excitement of realising this ambition, and becoming immersed in an incredibly intellectually rigorous and stimulating environment, inevitably promotes the desire to share knowledge with others.

Teaching and learning are complex processes, and the variety of skills used and resources available sometimes seem overwhelming to students. We feel, however, that face-to-face consultation and examination remain the bedrock of clinical examination, and are the fundamental skills required to practise medicine.

Students of paediatrics, whether undergraduate or postgraduate, medical or allied professional, general practitioner, general paediatrician, or system specialist, relate to patients by learning clinical examination techniques. Once the concepts are grasped by observing and practising oneself, the rewards of resolving clinical problems are legion.

Self-criticism and formal examination are paramount in the maintenance of standards and accountability; however, the main purpose of producing this resource is to share with you the expertise that specialist paediatricians use in their day-to-day practice, and also the fun and joy they experience in so doing.

You will observe by video the structured way in which each practitioner attempts to acquire important elements of medical history from child and parent, and augment this by examination of children of varying age. It is clear, particularly in the field of paediatrics, that flexibility is required in the art of both questioning and examination. One of the most useful things to do when revising and practising for a clinical exam is to observe others, and reflect on what you have seen. Fallibilities may be exhibited, and are part and parcel of life, but the important elements should not be overlooked. Not every condition can (or should) be covered in a resource such as this. We hope that we have been able to demonstrate a variety of problems seen in paediatrics, and that after watching the videos you will be able to formulate an approach that is transferable to a child or young person with any condition.

The text amplifies elements of the video clips, in particular focusing on the intellectual processes involved in decision-making, and will hopefully assist both the trainee undertaking formal examination and the experienced clinician faced with a diagnostic dilemma. We hope that you will learn from and enjoy the material as much as we have enjoyed collating it.

Paediatrics is a privilege. Advising parents about illness management is never easy and depends on the clinician understanding a number of factors. Knowledge of the subject matter is something that takes years to acquire and never ceases to confound and stimulate the enquiring mind. Acquiring knowledge is down to the individual and their learning style, yet listening and observing are paramount characteristics of the astute clinician. This book will, hopefully, be a facilitator of such skills, and will act as a seed to interest readers in the importance of sharing such knowledge and skills through medical education, as much as applying what is learnt, and not just in order to pass an examination.

In this technological era, it is often the case that information is mistaken for knowledge, and the sensitive clinician will make that distinction and have awareness and self-critique. The contributors to this project have all been chosen because of their personal attributes as much as their expertise, and it is those qualities that have made the journey in producing this work so enjoyable and that make multidisciplinary working such a joy within the specialty. The fundamental importance of history-taking and examination techniques in medicine remain the same as they have always been, and to see experts in action is something that is often undervalued by trainees and colleagues. We hope that this book in some way demonstrates our appreciation for colleagues and will act as a stimulant to others to develop their own skills.

We are indebted to the generous contributions of our colleagues at Alder Hey Children's NHS Foundation Trust and Royal Manchester Children's Hospital in this venture.

Mark and Ian

About the companion website

This book is accompanied by a companion website:

www.wiley.com/go/dalzell/paediatrics

Scan this QR code to visit the companion website:

The website features Clinical videos.

Chapter 1 **Rules of engagement (with the clinical examination and the examiners)**

Richard E. Appleton

The clinical examination and the examiners are now far better structured, prepared, and significantly more objective than even a decade ago. For each examination, the examiners' performance is critically evaluated both for consistency of the marks they award all the candidates in the station they examine and for consistency with their fellow examiners for each candidate. However, examiners, like candidates, are human and will, on occasions, be subject to their own idiosyncrasies and the effect of their environment, such as the phases of the moon, background radiation, and blood sugar level. With this in mind, the following guidance should help to prepare you for, and minimise the effects of, these unforeseen 'examiner moments'.

Do

- Be prepared.
- Be smartly dressed. Ties are unnecessary, and short sleeves are more acceptable and more comfortable for you to examine in.
- As soon as you enter the examination room/cubicle/bay – use your eyes and ears before 'hands on'.
- Be polite and courteous.
- Know – and show you know – how to talk with children.

Clinical Examination Skills in Paediatrics: For MRCPCH Candidates and Other Practitioners, First Edition. Edited by A. Mark Dalzell and Ian Sinha.
© 2020 John Wiley & Sons Ltd. Published 2020 by John Wiley & Sons Ltd.
Companion website: www.wiley.com/go/dalzell/paediatrics

- Even 20–30 seconds talking with the child will demonstrate to the examiner that you are treating the child as a person, not an object to be examined. It will also help you to establish a rapport with the child – which may prove very helpful for the rest of the examination.
- In the day(s) before you sit the examination think of topics of conversation that might help you to establish a rapport with the child.
- Do what the examiner asks in terms of a running commentary during your examination. If the examiner specifically asks for a running commentary as you examine the child – then do as the examiner asks! If the examiner doesn't specify – then do whatever you feel more comfortable doing.
- In the Communication station – remember, remember, remember: it is a dialogue and not a monologue. Listen to the role-player; ensure they understand what it is you will do, and then do this during the nine-minute station. Check that the role-player has understood what you have discussed with them as you proceed and certainly before the two-minute warning. If you can use diagrams/drawings to better communicate the specific topic – then do so.
- Allow time for summing up and discussion (with the examiner; with the role-player in the Communication scenarios); this should be no later than the two-minute warning in the clinical station as the final two minutes should be for the examiner to ask you questions on your findings – including the differential diagnosis, investigations, and management.
- Be honest. If you don't know an answer, be truthful and don't try to blag/waffle/lie as this will be more detrimental to your mark than saying, 'I'm sorry, I don't know.'
- Be confident but not arrogant.

Do not

- Wear dirty, badly creased, or threadbare clothes or shoes – it gives the wrong impression.
- Wear dresses/blouses with low necklines or gaping buttons – it certainly will give the wrong impression.
- Ignore the child as you examine them – or their parent/carer.
- Be rude to the child or their parent/carer.
- Be rude to, or aggressively challenge, an examiner.
- Force the child to co-operate.
- Make up signs that aren't there.
- Cheat (text/phone your mates before/after your examination to share scenarios etc.). This is immoral and carries a heavy penalty.

Chapter 2 **Tips for the communication station**

Andrew Riordan

This station is not really testing your knowledge – that's tested in other parts of the exam. This station tests your ability to communicate. The standard the examiner is looking for is that of a 'competent registrar'. Most of the marks are given for the way you say things, rather than what you say.

The station runs as follows.

Read the scenario

Before you enter the room you get the chance to read about the scenario. Read it carefully, then read it again. Think about what sort of scenario it is: explanation or negotiation.

Enter the room

There are three people in the room: the examiner, a 'parent', and you.

The examiner
The examiner introduces you to the 'parent' and then sits in the corner writing on the mark sheet. The examiner is unlikely to do anything else.

The 'parent'
The 'parent' may be a real parent, an actor, or a member of the hospital staff. They have a long list of questions that they want

Clinical Examination Skills in Paediatrics: For MRCPCH Candidates and Other Practitioners, First Edition. Edited by A. Mark Dalzell and Ian Sinha.
© 2020 John Wiley & Sons Ltd. Published 2020 by John Wiley & Sons Ltd.
Companion website: www.wiley.com/go/dalzell/paediatrics

you to answer. They may have a particular thing that they want to ask about.

You

Take a breath, relax, and go for it.

Introduction

Say 'My name is …' and describe your role from the scenario ('I am the paediatric registrar on call').

Check who the 'parent' is, and agree the aim of the scenario ('You wanted to talk about …' or 'What was it you wanted to talk to me about?').

Let the 'parent' ask their questions

There are broadly two types of scenario.

Explanation

Try to give a clear explanation without jargon. Find out what the 'parent' knows already and check they understand what you've said. Check if there's something else that they want to know ('Is there anything else you wanted to ask about?').

Negotiation

Try to explore the 'parent's' feelings and concerns. Use an appropriate questioning style ('Is there any particular reason why you don't want this treatment?').

Some scenarios may include safeguarding (refusing treatment), ethics (asking for inappropriate tests), or clinical incidents (drug errors).

Respond to the questions

Try to establish a rapport with the 'parent' – treat them like a 'normal human being'. Show empathy and respect ('This must be very difficult for you').

Chapter 2

Give information

The information you give needs to be accurate and appropriate for the questions the 'parent' has asked. Don't just give a nine-minute lecture on the subject.

Two minutes to go

When the 'two minutes to go' signal comes, use this as a cue to summarise your discussion and check understanding.

Time up

Thank the 'parent', say goodbye to the examiner, and move on to the next station.

Highlights
- Introduction
- Agree topic
- Ask what they know and what they want to know
- Answer clearly without jargon
- Check understanding
- Summarise

Chapter 2

Chapter 3 **Translating into medical-speak**

Daniel B. Hawcutt and Ian Sinha

When we talk about medical-speak, we mean the words doctors use to describe the symptoms, signs, procedures, etc. experienced by patients. Medical-speak is not there to obfuscate, or to elevate doctors from the public through the hiding of simple facts in obscure words. Rather, the language of medicine is there to convey very precise meanings, which mean the same to everyone who uses it. Everyday language lacks the precision and reproducibility of medical-speak. However, the translation into medical-speak *is* difficult at first. By the time you do your clinical exam, you should be able to understand what a patient is telling you and accurately translate it into medical-speak for your colleagues. In addition, you need to be able to un-translate, and communicate effectively with patients using appropriate lay terms. There are some common problems, however.

Problem 1: Pseudo-medical-speak

The general public will try and be helpful by using medical-sounding words when they talk to you. They genuinely believe they are using them correctly, but you cannot trust them. You have been taught to use open questions when taking a history. Generally this is good. However, when you are presented with medical(ish) terminology by a lay person, it is necessary to close

Clinical Examination Skills in Paediatrics: For MRCPCH Candidates and Other Practitioners, First Edition. Edited by A. Mark Dalzell and Ian Sinha.
© 2020 John Wiley & Sons Ltd. Published 2020 by John Wiley & Sons Ltd.
Companion website: www.wiley.com/go/dalzell/paediatrics

the questions down to establish exactly what they mean. Don't be afraid of asking very simple questions about whatever they are describing. The patient may not know exactly what symptom or procedure they had but they can usually give you a few clues. To be fair, it is not the patient's fault. Your job is to translate their words into the *correct* terminology.

The main categories of pseudo-medical-speak, to which you must be alert during any history, are as follows.

Fictional or ambiguous procedures

If a patient has had an operation or procedure, make sure it is what they say. If you have never heard of it, be doubly careful. One example might be a child who has had a 'bronchography'. In our experience this has been used by patients to mean a bronchogram, bronchoscopy, spirometry, upper gastrointestinal endoscopy, and MRI of the chest. It is your job is to ask exactly what happened, how they were afterwards, who did it …; in essence, anything you can to figure out what this procedure or investigation was.

Inappropriate symptom attribution

An excellent example of this is wheeze. Wheeze is a common symptom that patients will give for virtually any irregularity in breathing. They may be right, but never accept it at face value. Was it a high-pitched whistling noise? Was the noise on breathing in or out, or both? Did it get better with their inhaler? Best of all, make wheeze, stridor, and snoring noises in front of them and ask which they mean. Another example is the child with 'fits'. As you know, the child could be having any number of movement disorders, funny turns, or syncopal attacks.

Colloquialisms

Some of these are nationally recognisable – such as 'nervous breakdown', which can mean anything from a psychotic episode to a temper tantrum, while in paediatrics we commonly find children with septic tonsillitis or double pneumonia. There are also local variations, for example 'ruttles' in the chest that seem most prominent in Nottinghamshire. Find out what people mean, and if you are not 100% certain then ask more questions to find out exactly what they mean. Closed questions to establish the details are essential: Did you see your GP or a hospital doctor/psychiatrist? Did you need any treatment? What was it? How long did it last?

Problem 2: Using both types of speak at once (plain English and medical)

You will probably have been on lots of touchy–feely communication sessions so you can effectively talk and listen. This is undoubtedly a good thing for doctor–patient communication, as it means we can now explain to patients what is wrong with them in everyday English. It is also well worth trying to be good at too, as good communicators are much less likely to be sued or make catastrophic mistakes. However, because of the imprecision and non-reproducibility, it is rubbish for doctor–doctor communication. It lengthens the story unnecessarily, reduces clarity, and sounds amateurish. None of these will help you in the exam.

Once you begin to use medical-speak, there is usually a phase of double-speak. You will repeat yourself by saying in normal English what you have just said in medical.

An example may help show the difference:

Double-speak: *Jim was diagnosed with asthma, which can make it hard to breath. He was given some medicine, salbutamol, to relax his lungs, using an inhaler.*

Accurate medical-speak: *Mr Taylor was admitted with an exacerbation of asthma, requiring inhaled salbutamol.*

Double-speak can be excellent if talking to a patient, but will just frustrate your peers and examiners. The best way to overcome it is practice, and the more you present the better you will be.

In your exam you may come across patients with complex disorders that you may not understand completely. A general

Chapter 3

rule is to avoid using a medical term if you do not know what it means – you will use it incorrectly, and you will look foolish. Despite all that has gone before in this chapter, it is better to use the simpler, non-medical term if you are confused or in doubt. But by practising, you will learn more and this situation will rapidly disappear.

Top tip

Some words are used badly by a lot of doctors too. However, it pays to learn to use them the right way for when the curmudgeonly old examiner who actually gives a damn about use of language turns up. The most common example here is nauseous/nauseated. Someone who feels sick is *nauseated*. Something that makes you feel sick is *nauseous*.

For example: Mary found the smell of vomit nauseous. After her sister had been sick, the smell lingered and she became nauseated.

In 99% of cases it will not matter if you use nauseous for either or both, but for that one occasion it will make you shine.

Highlights
- Always
  - try to establish exactly what the patient means; use closed questions if necessary
  - translate the history (except the presenting complaint) into medical-speak as best you can.
- Never
  - repeat yourself by using medical-speak followed by plain English
  - use lay words or descriptions when you do not know what they mean.

Chapter 4 **Cardiovascular examination**

Michael T. Bowes and Caroline B. Jones

Key points to consider while conducting your examination

- Is there evidence of cyanosis or heart failure?
- Are there any signs of an associated chromosomal or genetic disease?
- Does the child appear to be failing to thrive?
- Are there any scars suggestive of previous heart surgery?

Positioning the child

Position babies flat in a cot wearing just a nappy, and toddlers on a parent's lap. Ideally, position older children on the couch at 45° with the chest entirely exposed (although not for adolescent girls).

From the end of the bed

- Is the child comfortable?
  - Look for signs of increased work of breathing.
  - Count the respiratory rate.
- Is the child dysmorphic? In particular, for a cardiovascular examination:
  - trisomy 21 (atrioventricular septal defect, ventricular and atrial septal defects)

Clinical Examination Skills in Paediatrics: For MRCPCH Candidates and Other Practitioners, First Edition. Edited by A. Mark Dalzell and Ian Sinha.
© 2020 John Wiley & Sons Ltd. Published 2020 by John Wiley & Sons Ltd.
Companion website: www.wiley.com/go/dalzell/paediatrics

- Turner syndrome (left-sided heart lesions, coarctation of the aorta)
  - 22q11 deletion (conotruncal abnormalities, common arterial trunk, interruption of the aorta, tetralogy of Fallot)
  - Williams syndrome (supravalvular aortic stenosis, peripheral pulmonary artery stenosis)
  - Noonan syndrome (valvular pulmonary stenosis).
- Extra clues
  - Does the child have a nasogastric or percutaneous gastrostomy (PEG) tube to supplement feeding?
  - Other features that may help you to identify an underlying syndrome, e.g.
  - limb abnormalities in association with Holt–Oram syndrome
  - eye signs such as Brushfield spots in children with trisomy 21
  - cleft lip and palate repair scar
  - arachnodactyly or high arched palate in Marfan syndrome.
  - Does the child require supplementary oxygen?
- Is the child appropriately grown?
  - Infants who appear small for their age, or older children with short stature, may have chronic disease, heart failure, or a syndrome.
  - Tall stature may signify Marfan syndrome.

Important signs to look for (and not miss)

- Hands – peripheral perfusion and palmar creases. In older children, check for clubbing and stigmata of bacterial endocarditis.
- Cyanosis – peripheral/central (often noted on the bridge of the nose in infants).
- Assess brachial pulse rate and rhythm for 10 seconds (leave femoral pulses until the end, but don't forget to palpate them!).

- Apex beat – may be in the 4th intercostal space in children under four years. Remember that dextrocardia is frequently encountered in exams.
- Heaves and thrills. Note that heaves can be difficult to distinguish in young children with an active praecordium.
- Jugular venous pulse (JVP) should not be performed in children under four years, but consider it in older children with heart failure and in teenagers.
- Palpate the liver edge. This is usually palpable in children under four years. Percussion can be helpful to locate the upper edge.

What scars might you see?

- Cardiac surgical scars – left or right thoracotomy, median sternotomy.
- Smaller scars – chest drains, central lines, cardiac catheterisation, gastrostomy, or abdominal pacemaker.

Heart sounds and murmurs

- Listen over all five areas (remember the back) with the diaphragm, whilst palpating the pulse, then repeat at the apex with the bell.
- Radiation can be difficult to elicit in babies, but consider it in toddlers at the end of auscultation. If you hear a murmur at the upper sternal edge listen at the carotid for radiation. If the murmur is best heard at the apex move the child to the left lateral decubitus position and auscultate the axilla.
- In infants, attempt to repeat the process in a different position to detect postural variation (particularly if you suspect an innocent murmur).
- Heart sounds:
  - most commonly heart sounds will be 'normal with a...'
  - prosthetic metallic heart sounds should be easily identifiable
  - only comment on abnormal sounds such as 'wide splitting of the second heart sound' if you are confident in your findings

Chapter 4

- abnormal heart sounds are rarely identifiable in younger children with fast heart rates.
- Murmurs should be described according to the:
  - intensity or volume – graded 1–6/6 systolic and 1–4/4 diastolic
  - timing in the cardiac cycle
    - systolic – ejection, pansystolic
    - diastolic – early, mid, or late (though this may be difficult)
    - continuous
    - most murmurs in infancy will be systolic or continuous
  - site at which they are heard maximally (loud murmurs are often heard throughout the praecordium, particularly in infants, but you should state where you think they are loudest)
  - radiation.

Additional components of the cardiovascular examination

- Measure the blood pressure and oxygen saturation.
- Plot the child's height and weight on a centile chart.
- Listen to the lung bases – you are unlikely to have a child with pulmonary oedema attending the examination, but this gives you valuable time to gather your thoughts.
- Palpate the ankles to look for oedema.
- Check for radio-femoral delay in teenagers.

How to summarise your findings

'From my examination, I have found that _____

- is comfortable at rest/has some increased work of breathing
- is pink/has signs of central cyanosis
- has no scars/describe scars
- has heart sounds that are normal/abnormal …
- … with a murmur (describe)/no murmur.'

Questions to prepare

- Consider which investigations you require to make a complete assessment.
- You should know common genetic or chromosomal abnormalities associated with congenital heart disease.
- Be able to list common lesions presenting with either cyanosis or heart failure in the neonate.
- Be able to suggest operations that the child may have undergone.
- Be aware of treatments for infants with heart failure (typically left to right shunt) and failure to thrive – including medications and nutritional support.

Top tips

- Stick with the brachial pulses as they are most reliable in all ages.
- Pedal pulses may be a less intrusive way of gaining information, prior to femoral palpation (but not instead of).
- Look thoroughly for scars, especially thoracotomy scars, which often can't be seen from the front. When examining adolescent girls, who should leave their bra on, ask if they have any scars underneath.
- Palpate for the apex beat on both sides together initially.
- You should be able to combine palpation for heaves and thrills with three hand movements and the suprasternal notch.
- If you hear a murmur palpate the area of maximal intensity again after auscultation to be certain there isn't an accompanying thrill.
- Repeating the auscultation process in a different position at the end of the examination will allow you to detect postural variation and give you another chance to confirm your findings prior to presentation.
- Reaching a diagnosis following a cardiovascular examination is often difficult (and in reality often requires an

Chapter 4

echocardiogram), so present in a logical structured fashion and don't jump straight to the diagnosis.

Possible scenarios

In the child without scars:

- Your main focus will be correctly identifying the murmur.
- The examiner will expect you to suggest a diagnosis.
- *Example*: 'As _____ has some evidence of increased work of breathing and a pansystolic murmur at the left lower sternal edge I suspect she has a ventricular septal defect or perhaps an atrioventricular septal defect.'
- *Example*: 'As _____ has a 3/6 ejection systolic murmur at the right upper sternal edge that radiates to the carotids, I suspect he has aortic stenosis.'

In the child with surgical scars and cyanosis or evidence of heart failure:

- These children are likely to have complex congenital heart disease and undergone surgical 'palliative' procedures rather than complete repair.
- They may or may not have a murmur – this is unlikely to help you make a diagnosis.
- *Example*: 'As _____ is cyanosed and has a midline sternotomy scar I suspect that she has had palliative surgery for complex congenital heart disease. This is likely to be a univentricular type of circulation such as hypoplastic left heart syndrome.'
- Making a definitive diagnosis will be difficult but you should at least present a logical thought process.

In the child with surgical scars and *no* cyanosis or evidence of heart failure:

- These children are likely to have had surgical repair, though may have residual lesions or murmurs.
- A murmur may be helpful in making a diagnosis, but other clues such as signs of an associated syndrome may be more helpful to suggest the underlying heart problem.
- *Example:* 'As _____ appears well with no evidence of cyanosis or heart failure I suspect she has repaired congenital heart disease. She has a median sternotomy scar, and findings consistent with trisomy 21, so I suspect she has had closure of a septal defect in the past.'
- *Example:* 'As _____ appears well with no evidence of cyanosis or heart failure I suspect he has repaired congenital heart disease. He has a median sternotomy scar, a 2/6 pulmonary murmur, and findings consistent with 22q11 deletion. This would lead me to suspect he has a repair for tetralogy of Fallot and may have residual pulmonary stenosis.'
- *Example*: 'As _____ appears well with no evidence of cyanosis or heart failure I suspect she has repaired congenital heart disease. She has signs consistent with Turner syndrome and a lateral thoracotomy scar so I suspect that she has had a repair of coarctation in the past.'
- *Example:* 'As _____ appears well with no evidence of cyanosis or heart failure I suspect he has had surgical correction of congenital heart disease. He has a median sternotomy scar, a 2/6 pan-systolic murmur at the apex, and also has findings consistent with trisomy 21. This would lead me to suspect he has had a repair of an atrioventricular septal defect and may have some residual mitral valve regurgitation.'

Chapter 4

Chapter 5 **Respiratory examination**

Anna Shawcross and Sarah J. Mayell

Key points to consider while conducting your examination

- Whether there is evidence of chronic respiratory illness.
- Whether the child is currently well, or has increased work of breathing.
- Whether the child has any evidence of other conditions predisposing him or her to respiratory disease.

Positioning the child

When examining infants, you will gain far more useful information if they are settled and happy, rather than cross and crying! They are likely to be happiest on a parent's knee, so examine them there rather than on a couch. Ideally, position older children on the couch at 45° with the chest entirely exposed (although not for adolescent girls).

From the end of the bed

- Is the child comfortable?
  - Count the respiratory rate.
  - Spend time looking for signs of increased work of breathing: nasal flaring; tracheal tug; subcostal/intercostal recession.

Clinical Examination Skills in Paediatrics: For MRCPCH Candidates and Other Practitioners, First Edition. Edited by A. Mark Dalzell and Ian Sinha.
© 2020 John Wiley & Sons Ltd. Published 2020 by John Wiley & Sons Ltd.
Companion website: www.wiley.com/go/dalzell/paediatrics

- If you hear a noise at this point, comment on it, e.g. stridor, cough (and, if present, whether it sounds wet/dry).
- Is the child dysmorphic? In particular, for a respiratory examination:
  - trisomy 21 (upper airway problems, cardiac problems, recurrent infections)
  - connective tissue disorders predisposing to pneumothorax (e.g. Ehlers–Danlos or Marfan syndrome)
  - cushingoid features suggestive of long-term steroid use.
- Clues around the bed:
  - Supplementary oxygen/monitoring?
  - Any medications (e.g. inhaler with spacer, pancreatic enzyme supplements)?
  - Does the child have a nasogastric tube or gastrostomy? This would suggest a chronic problem requiring nutritional support (e.g. cystic fibrosis or chronic lung disease of prematurity) or difficulty with swallowing.
  - Does the child have intravenous access? An infant is unlikely to have a long-term access device such as a port-a-cath (which may well be seen in the examination of an older child) but may have another access device.
  - Is there evidence of another underlying condition? For example, neurological or neuromuscular conditions, or an appearance suggestive of prematurity.
- Is the child appropriately grown?

Important signs to look for (and not miss)

- Clubbing – not usually present <1 year.
- Central and peripheral cyanosis.
- Chest wall abnormality/asymmetry – inspect from both the front and side.
- Checking the mediastinal position by palpating for the apex beat (this should ensure you don't miss dextrocardia, which might signify primary ciliary dyskinesia) and gentle palpation of the trachea.

What scars might you see?

- Pay particular attention to the back and underarms for chest drain and thoracotomy scars, and to the neck for central line scars suggestive of Paediatric Intensive Care Unit admission.
- An abdominal scar in a child with cystic fibrosis may be from surgery for meconium ileus.

Auscultation

Listen throughout the chest, anteriorly then posteriorly, for

- crackles
- wheeze
- transmitted sounds from the upper airway (these are common in infants, particularly those with underlying neurological problems).

Additional components of the respiratory examination

- ENT examination: this is the start of the respiratory tract.
- If your findings suggest it would be relevant, say you would like to examine the abdomen or cardiovascular system.
- In older children say you would measure peak flow, and inspect a sputum sample. Remember, however, that these cannot be routinely performed in infants (unless you have access to specialised equipment!) and are unlikely to produce sputum, so avoid saying you would like to ask for these.

How to summarise your findings

'From my examination, I have found that _____

- does/does not have some increased work of breathing
- does/does not have (… relevant clues suggestive of underlying diagnoses or chronic illness, such as dysmorphism, supplemental O_2, scars)
- does/does not have adequate nutritional status.'

Then describe your auscultation findings:

- are there equal breath sounds throughout the chest?
- are there added sounds (and where did you hear them)?

Questions to prepare

- What are the causes of bronchiectasis?
- What might you expect to see on a chest radiograph of this child?
- What might you see on spirometry?
- What are the side effects of long-term steroid use?

Top tips

- Don't percuss aimlessly and endlessly.
- When feeling the apex beat with your right hand, feel the trachea with your left and then count down – this looks slick.
- Tailoring the examination for infants:
  - The role of palpation is limited – in reality, you will find that you move quite quickly from observation to auscultation and come back to palpation as necessary. This should ensure you don't miss the window for auscultation in a wary infant.
  - Percussion is likely to upset an infant and should only be performed if indicated.
  - Observation of chest wall movement may well suffice, rather than measuring chest expansion.

Possible scenarios

You may come across children with varying degrees of chronic respiratory illness, reflecting the diversity of this specialty. Some examples you may come across include:

- A child with cystic fibrosis – the clues pointing towards this diagnosis include medications around the bed, central venous access, clubbing, hyperinflation, and widespread crackles or wheeze. Remember that these may be absent, however.

- A child with localised auscultation findings who may be otherwise well – consider localised bronchiectasis, intercurrent infection, or a structural lung problem.
- A child with an underlying neurological disorder (see Chapter 6).
- A child with several scars on the chest – these may be from chest drains for recurrent pneumothoraces.

Chapter 6 **Respiratory examination in a child with neurodisability**

Clare P. Halfhide

Key points to consider while conducting your examination

- How severe is the neurodisability? Think about the GMFCS score (Gross Motor Function Classification System score 1–5).
- Is there evidence of chronic respiratory illness?
- Is the child currently well?
- Are the findings localised or generalised in the chest?
- Has this respiratory diagnosis predisposed the child to other problems (e.g. pulmonary hypertension, failure to thrive, liver disease), or have the child's other problems (e.g. scoliosis or direct aspiration from eating) predisposed him or her to respiratory issues?

Positioning the child

- It is important to ascertain from the parent or carer *before you start* how the child with severe neurodisability indicates if they are happy or upset. Laughter does not always indicate happiness.
- If a child is wheelchair dependent it may be useful to examine him or her both in the wheelchair and on a bed as a child's breathing pattern can significantly alter in a range of positions,

Clinical Examination Skills in Paediatrics: For MRCPCH Candidates and Other Practitioners, First Edition. Edited by A. Mark Dalzell and Ian Sinha.
© 2020 John Wiley & Sons Ltd. Published 2020 by John Wiley & Sons Ltd.
Companion website: www.wiley.com/go/dalzell/paediatrics

and can affect quality of life (e.g. attending school). This may not be possible if hoisting equipment is unavailable, but you should suggest it.

- Do not distress the child. Always ask about the most comfortable position in which to examine him or her.

From the end of the bed

The initial general inspection is *key* to respiratory examination of the child with neurodisability.

- How severe is the child's neurodisability?
  - What is the overall motor function of the child? Is the child wheelchair dependent?
  - What is the overall tone of the child's head and trunk? Is it reduced or increased? Is there dystonia present?
  - How does the child control oral secretions? Does the child mouth breath or drool?
  - Is there scoliosis, which may cause restrictive lung disease?
  - Ask the child to cough. If they are able to, does it seem effective?
- Is the child comfortable?
  - Note the position that the child is in and if they appear comfortable. For example, in a wheelchair, on a bed on one side, neck hyperextended?
  - Does the child require supplemental oxygen? If so, how much?
  - Count the respiratory rate. Note any evidence of abnormal central respiratory drive with breath-holding or central apnoeas. Often children with neurodisability can become dystonic or breath-hold when examined for the first time by a stranger.
  - Are there signs of increased work of breathing?
  - Look for paradoxical breathing.

- Extra clues
  - Are there hyoscine patches behind the ears (or rarely between the scapulae)? Are there any medications/equipment around the bed?
  - Does the child have a gastrostomy? Consider that the child may have difficulty swallowing, or may require supplementary nutrition.
  - Oxygen saturation monitor, portable suction, oxygen cylinders or concentrator, mask ventilator?
  - Does the child have a tracheostomy?
- Is the child appropriately grown?

Important signs to look for (and not miss)

- Is there clubbing? This is rare but may indicate bronchiectasis.
- Is there central cyanosis? In some children with neurodisability we do not aim to achieve saturations >93%. Note if this is in oxygen.
- Note the upper airway shape, i.e. the size of the jaw and tongue.
- Is there any evidence of upper airway obstruction, i.e. stridor or suprasternal recession? Does repositioning affect this obstructed breathing pattern? Is there a tracheostomy?
- Is there a port-a-cath? This is usually placed in the subclavicular area but can also be put in the mid-axillary line or abdominally. Remember that these might only be identified on palpation.
- Is there any evidence of spinal surgery?
- Is there an intrathecal baclofen pump in situ?
- Note the chest shape and presence of scoliosis? Do both sides of the chest look an equal size?
- Apex beat and tracheal position – mediastinal shift due to scoliosis is common (and dextrocardia is common in exams).
- Is there a dull percussion note?

What scars might you see?

- Are there neck scars from central lines, thoracotomy scars, or spinal scars?
- Previous port-a-cath scars

Chest auscultation

- Are there added upper airway sounds? It is acceptable to ask for the tracheostomy to be suctioned if needed.
- Listen in upper/mid- and lower zones on both front and back. Also auscultate in the apices and supraclavicular areas. Are the breath sounds vesicular throughout the lung fields or not?
- Are there added sounds, and are these localised or generalised?
  - Coarser crackles are likely to be due to fluid or secretions in the airway; finer crackles could be either interstitial lung disease or pulmonary oedema.
  - Wheeze suggests airway narrowing, either from asthma or from secretions.

Additional components of the respiratory examination in a child with underlying neurological problems

These can be remembered using the acronym PACES:

- Peak flow/spirometry (if the child is able to). Spirometry is a very crude test as a one-off measurement. You might suggest doing lying and sitting forced vital capacity to look for diaphragmatic weakness, or cough peak flow if you suspect a neuromuscular problem.
- Abdominal examination (in particular to look for hepatomegaly).
- Cardiovascular examination to look for pulmonary hypertension (loud, split S2).
- ENT examination with the correct equipment (including inspection of the nasal passages).
- Sputum examination (in an older child).

How to summarise your findings

'From my examination, I have found that _____

- is/is not wheelchair bound, and has increased/decreased tone (this must be done sensitively)
- is comfortable at rest/has some increased work of breathing/ needs oxygen/has scoliosis
- does/does not have signs suggestive of chronic respiratory illness such as … (state what the positive findings are)
- does/does not have vesicular breathing throughout the lung fields, and does/does not have added sounds (describe them).'

Questions to prepare

- What are the main causes of respiratory infection in children with neurodisability? These include immobility, direct aspiration, reflux aspiration, poor cough, seizures, and recurrent infections.
- What are the causes of bronchiectasis?
- How does scoliosis affect respiratory function?

Top tips

- Don't be thrown off track because the child has neurological problems. You will have seen children like this frequently, and your approach just needs to be logical and thorough.
- Be sensitive and respectful, as you would with any patient, and engage as much as possible with the child.
- Before moving any part of the child's body, ask if this will cause pain.

Possible scenarios

Children with various neurological diagnoses develop respiratory complications. In particular, you may be asked to examine a child with cerebral palsy, or one with neuromuscular weakness.

Chapter 6

Chapter 7 **Gastrointestinal examination**

Anastasia Konidari and A. Mark Dalzell

Key points to consider while conducting your examination

- Is the child currently well?
- Is there evidence of acute or chronic gastrointestinal (GI) illness?
- Is the child jaundiced?
- Does the child have stigmata of liver disease?
- Are there any abdominal masses? In particular does the child have hepatomegaly, splenomegaly, or both?
- Does the child have a multisystem disorder that affects the GI system or nutritional status (e.g. cystic fibrosis, cerebral palsy, tumour, renal failure, or metabolic disease)?
- Has the child's illness affected other systems, or is the child at risk of additional comorbidities (e.g. protein calorie malnutrition, infections, delayed puberty, endocrinopathy, increased risk of malignancies)?

Positioning the child

Expose the child's abdomen from the nipples to the knees, but keep underwear on. Maintain the child's dignity at all times, using blankets if needed. Lie the child as flat as possible.

Clinical Examination Skills in Paediatrics: For MRCPCH Candidates and Other Practitioners, First Edition. Edited by A. Mark Dalzell and Ian Sinha.
© 2020 John Wiley & Sons Ltd. Published 2020 by John Wiley & Sons Ltd.
Companion website: www.wiley.com/go/dalzell/paediatrics

From the end of the bed

- Is the child comfortable or in pain?
- Is the child jaundiced or pale? If possible, assess these in natural daylight.
- Is there abdominal distension, protruding masses, or scars?
- Look for rashes – especially an eczematous patch or erythema nodosum.
- Note the nutritional status.
- Note the presence of telangiectasias or spider naevi.
- Relevant dysmorphism:
  - syndrome predisposing to GI pathology (trisomy 21, Alagille syndrome, Zellweger spectrum disorder)
  - pigmented lesions on the lips and face (Peutz–Jeghers syndrome)
  - cushingoid appearance (consider long-term steroid use in inflammatory bowel disease).
- Extra clues
  - Does the child have a gastrostomy, nasal feeding tube, or a stoma?
  - Are there any venous ports or intravenous access (for parenteral nutrition)?
  - Does the child use any medications, infant formula, or special feeds, or a wheelchair?

Important signs to look for (and not miss)

- Jaundice, cyanosis, or pallor.
- Clubbing.
- Stigmata of liver disease, including palmar erythema, telangiectasias, or koilonychia.
- Oedema (may signify severe malnutrition).
- Muscle wasting or significantly decreased subcutaneous fat.
- Joint swelling (inflammatory bowel disease).
- Abdominal distension.
- Abdominal tenderness.

- Presence, and quality, of bowel sounds.
- Stomas.

What scars might you see?

- Kocher incision in the region of the liver = hepatic surgery.
- Laparotomy scars (mid-line or paramedian) imply major abdominal surgery.
- Small scars on the lateral aspect of the abdomen may be the result of peritoneal dialysis.
- Scar in the lower abdomen may be a result of renal transplant.
- Gastrostomies (epigastric), ileostomies (right iliac fossa), colostomies (left iliac fossa).

Abdominal examination

- During palpation (superficial and deep), be gentle, caring, and try not to cause discomfort.
- Examine at the same level as the abdomen.
- Ask the child about discomfort or pain first.
- Look at the child's face during palpation, and ask the child to flex his or her knees to relax voluntary abdominal tension.
- Start from either the right or left iliac fossa, and palpate all four quadrants in turn.
- Note any hernias, masses, or organomegaly – start palpation in the right iliac fossa and synchronise palpation with the child's breathing. Bimanually examine both kidneys. Percuss the spleen and liver:
  - feeling a liver edge of one to two fingerbreadths below the right costal margin is normal in infants and younger children
  - a palpable spleen may be just palpable in infants, but should be considered abnormal.
- Remember to auscultate for bowel sounds and bruits.
- To test for ascites, examine for shifting dullness and fluid thrill (more difficult in infants or toddlers).

- Inform the examiner that you would ideally like to inspect the genitalia and anal area (including digital rectal examination if appropriate).

Additional components of the gastrointestinal examination

Ask to inspect stool and urine.

How to summarise your findings

'From my examination, I have found that _____

- is/is not comfortable at rest, does/does not have abdominal discomfort, and does/does not have abdominal distension
- does/does not have signs suggestive of chronic GI illness, e.g. …
- is thriving/malnourished/underweight for age/obese/thin
- does/does not have abdominal pain, organomegaly, abdominal mass, and the bowel sounds are … (describe the bowel sounds).'

  Expand on other systems if relevant.

Questions to prepare

- What are the main causes of faltering growth or severe weight loss?
- What are the causes of clubbing?
- What are the causes of jaundice?
- What are the common GI pathologies in different age groups?
- What are the causes of recurrent vomiting, blood in stool, severe abdominal pain?
- What will you see on abdominal radiographs in children with bowel perforation?
- Have a basic knowledge of types of infant formula and special feeds.
- What are the side effects of long-term corticosteroid use in growing children?

Chapter 7

Top tips

- If there is liver disease, think about fat-soluble vitamin malabsorption.
- Always emphasise the importance of providing adequate supplementation to the growing child.

Possible scenarios

- You should formulate. differential diagnoses for the child with hepatomegaly, splenomegaly, or hepatosplenomegaly (note the child may or may not be jaundiced).
- A child or young person with inflammatory bowel disease.
- A child with chronic constipation.

Chapter 8 Examining a child with a renal transplant

Dean Wallace

Renal transplantation is the current gold standard treatment of end-stage renal failure worldwide. It is a favourite of examiners because of the wealth of clinical signs, features, and scars.

Renal transplants are often performed in patients with end-stage renal failure, and on some modality of dialysis, but can be performed pre-emptively. The transplant can be from deceased donors (DDKT) or live-related donors/family members (LRDKT). Pending organ availability, the average waiting time is 3–18 months.

Key points to consider while conducting your examination

- Are there any identifying features of fluid balance, electrolyte homeostasis, blood pressure, bone metabolism, red blood cell production, acid–base balance, growth, and nutrition, as well as details of the transplant?
- Are there any signs which may give clues to the child's renal history and even aetiology? Consider how long the child was in end-stage renal failure, and how much were he or she was compromised.
- Are there features of immunosuppression?

Clinical Examination Skills in Paediatrics: For MRCPCH Candidates and Other Practitioners, First Edition. Edited by A. Mark Dalzell and Ian Sinha.
© 2020 John Wiley & Sons Ltd. Published 2020 by John Wiley & Sons Ltd.
Companion website: www.wiley.com/go/dalzell/paediatrics

Positioning the child

Try to examine infants while they are sitting on a parent's lap, and older children lying flat. If older children have pulmonary oedema, they may not find it comfortable to lie flat, so ask them first.

From the end of the bed

- Even from afar, start to ask yourself what kind of nutritional/ growth state the child may be in.
- Think about the child's fluid status – is the child oedematous?
- Paraphernalia around the bed may include home peritoneal dialysis machines, central line covers, PD fluid bags, etc.
- Does the child look dysmorphic? The child's renal condition might be part of a syndrome, such as those mentioned below.

Important signs to look for (and not miss)

- Look carefully at the child's hands for signs of anaemia.
- Look in the child's mouth for signs of anaemia, dental enamel hypoplasia, aphthous ulcers (side effects), and the hydration of the mucous membranes.
- Look for thickened wrists, rachitic rosary (renal rickets).
- Does the child have any hearing aids/deafness (think Alport syndrome) or pre-auricular pits/pinna defects (Treacher Collins syndrome)?
- Does the child have any visual problems, i.e. cataracts (cystinosis)?
- Hypertrichosis and gingival overgrowth may be a side effect of ciclosporin immunosuppression (rare choice these days).
- Look for any evidence of steroid side effects.
- Palpate both of the child's arms gently for the distinctive vibration and bruit of an arteriovenous fistula (used for haemodialysis).
- As you work your way down to the chest, look for any current central lines or evidence of previous scarring in those areas.
- Look at both the anterior and posterior aspects of the abdomen for scarring.

Chapter 8

- Absence of abdominal muscles = prune belly syndrome.
- Palpation
  - Note the presence of any ascites/indwelling PD fluid if a catheter is still present (the graft may be non-functioning or failing).
  - Palpate the graft – it should be non-tender and fairly immobile.
  - Don't forget to ballot for remaining native kidneys! Enlarged ballotable kidneys may be present in polycystic kidney disease (either autosomal recessive or dominant), multicystic dysplastic kidney, obstructed systems, and renal tumours.
  - Palpate specifically for the bladder, which may be enlarged and neurogenic.
- Percussion
  - Percuss the quadrants, as per normal examination. Flank dullness may reveal polycystic enlarged kidneys, an enlarged dull bladder, and even identify the graft location (if the scar isn't clue enough).
- Auscultation
  - As well as standard bowel sounds, auscultate directly over the graft to assess for bruits, which could indicate graft stenosis or traumatic arteriovenous fistulae post biopsy.
  - Also auscultate the areas of the renal vessels to assess for bruits related to the native kidneys. This is unlikely to be relevant, since renal artery stenosis severe enough to cause end-stage renal failure would have necessitated nephrectomies. However, the native kidneys may have been biopsied themselves previously.

What scars might you see?

- Transverse/linear 3–5 cm scars over the renal angles will probably represent previous nephrectomies.
- Curvilinear scars in the right/left lower abdomen are usually the transplant site scars. (The transplanted kidneys are placed very anteriorly – usually extraperitoneally – and anastomosed

Chapter 8

with the internal iliac vessels in small children, and external iliac vessels in larger children.)
- Peri-umbilical scars may be from old PD catheters.
- Look for PD catheters, which may still be there if the transplant was relatively recent. (They are thicker, larger, and more superiorly placed than suprapubic urinary catheters.)
- Look for ileal conduits/Mitrofanoff stomas, which may indicate that transplantation was necessary for abnormal nephro-uretero-vesical anatomy requiring diversion to relieve backpressure.
- The transplanted kidney may have been biopsied several times, thereby creating some smaller (<0.5 cm) scars around the region of the graft.

Additional components of the examination

- Blood pressure – preferably manual.
- Urinalysis – particularly for protein content.
- An assessment of the external genitalia for further clues.
- If the child is oedematous – the opportunity to perform a full cardiorespiratory examination and fluid balance assessment (i.e. jugular venous pulse [JVP] lung bases. etc.).

Top tips

- Remember that the child may have had more than one transplant!
- For extra points, comment on the presence or absence of warty lesions in the hands, which can happen in immunosuppression.
- Look at the legs (and outer thighs in particular) for signs of recurrent subcutaneous injections (i.e. erythropoietin or low molecular weight heparin).

Chapter 9 **Examining a child with cerebral palsy**

Rachel Kneen and Anand S. Iyer

Key points to consider while conducting your examination

- Is this a central or peripheral neurological problem?
- Is the child ambulant?
- If not ambulant, then how does the child achieve mobility?
- Review of the wheelchair/assisted devices, e.g. orthotics for mobility.
- Observe the child's social communication skills.

Positioning the child

- Remember to always introduce yourself to the child in a way you think they will understand. Talk to the child, even if communication skills are limited – parents like doctors who talk to their children. Check the child's understanding, and ask the parent to let you know if the child is uncomfortable or in pain.
- Tell the child and parent how you are going to perform the examination. For example, 'I am going to move your legs, can you please make them go all floppy like a jelly?'

Clinical Examination Skills in Paediatrics: For MRCPCH Candidates and Other Practitioners, First Edition. Edited by A. Mark Dalzell and Ian Sinha.
© 2020 John Wiley & Sons Ltd. Published 2020 by John Wiley & Sons Ltd.
Companion website: www.wiley.com/go/dalzell/paediatrics

From the end of the bed

- Observe the child's activities and play.
- Any facial dysmorphism, or neurocutaneous stigmata pointing to a possible genetic problem?
- Observe the child's speech. Is it clear or not? Is it repetitive?
- Does the child drool, or have any hyoscine patches behind the ear?
- Ask if the child is ambulant. Observe the child's gait (diplegic gait, scissoring, hemiplegic gait). Look for asymmetry – children with spastic diplegia often have one side more affected than the other.
- If the child uses walking aids or a wheelchair, note the details – electric powered, self-propelled, or attendant propelled. Also look for assisted devices like walking aids, tripod sticks, a K-walker, or a standing frame.
- Wheelchair – look for truncal and neck support, hand rails on the wheels pointing to predominantly lower limb problems, finger-triggered switch, whether the wheelchair can be made flat in the case of seizures.
- Any orthotic devices, such as an ankle–foot orthosis (AFO), pressure relief ankle–foot orthosis (PRAFO), wrist and hand splints, Lycra body suits for truncal stability? It helps if you know the names of these devices and can describe the details, e.g. is the AFO rigid or hinged.
- Does the child have a percutaneous gastrostomy (PEG) or nasogastric (NG) tube?
- Does the child have a tracheostomy or use supplementary oxygen or a suction machine?
- Does the child use a non-invasive ventilation device?
- Observe how the child communicates, and describe any problems.
- Note if the child is wearing nappies or an incontinence pad and comment if this is beyond the normal age you would expect this to be present.

Important signs to look for (and not miss)

- Look at the child's posture in the chair or while seated.
- Observe the child's gait, and ability to stand up from a seated position.
- In mild hemiplegic cerebral palsy, utilise other ways to elicit weakness:
  - The Fogg test is elicited by asking the child to walk on the heel or outside of the foot. Observe the upper limb posturing, which correlates with the side that is weak.
  - Ask the child to raise his or her arms and keep them on the same level, then ask the child to close his or her eyes. The side that is weak shows gradual pronation and falls down, this is called 'pronator drift'.
  - If the hemiplegia is obvious, doing these manoeuvres may cause the child to fall and get hurt, so do not do them for all cases.
- Look for calf, hamstring, and upper limb muscle atrophy due to disuse, and also neurovascular changes such as smooth skin, loss of hair, and lymphoedema.
- Look for any pumps inserted in the abdomen (intrathecal baclofen) – these give a circular-like swelling in the hip area.
- Contractures may be visible (predominantly elbow, knees, ankle).
- Look for ptosis, strabismus, or visual impairment (roving eyes).
- Assess the child's tone by passive movements across the joints, i.e. moving the ankle through dorsiflexion and plantarflexion passively, then doing the dorsiflexion quickly. Often this dynamic–passive movement would lead to a 'catch' in movement, which is what is described as 'clasp knife' rigidity seen classically in pyramidal lesions. 'Lead pipe' rigidity seen in parkinsonism is very rare in children. If not sure, you could say that there is increased tone in the muscle groups across the ankle. Note that in most children with spastic quadriplegic

cerebral palsy, there would be neck and truncal hypotonia and peripheral hypertonia.

- Power should be assessed formally in a communicative child. After the gait inspection, ask the child to move to the examination bed. In children with diplegia, start with the lower limbs; in those with hemiplegia, start from upper limbs. Give short, clear instructions and examine broad muscle groups. Grade the power using Medical Research Council (MRC) grading (1–5). Mentioning power is grade 5 in the upper limb is not specific – you will need to break it down as shoulder abductors, adductors, elbow flexors and extensors, wrist dorsiflexors and palmarflexors, etc. …. Or mention that power is broadly normal across all muscle groups. If the child is unwilling to cooperate but can walk, it is reasonable to say that the power must be at least 4 in all groups. A useful way of encouraging a child to cooperate is to turn the instructions into a game or competition, e.g. 'I bet you can't do X', 'can you kick my hand?' This shows you have examined children before.
- Intrinsic finger muscles, abductor pollicis brevis, and abductor digiti minimi are very specific muscle groups and are usually affected as a whole in pyramidal lesions – they have more diagnostic value in peripheral nerve lesions.
- In a non-communicative child, it can be difficult to formally assess power using the MRC status. Check with the examiner and parent if the child can be moved and examined in the bed or on the wheelchair. Start with observing the spontaneous movements and anti-gravity movements, and ask the parent about the abilities of the child; for example, whether the child is able to lift or bend his or her legs. Mention that it is difficult to formally assess power, but, from the wheelchair, observation of spontaneous movements, and discussion with the parent, it is likely that the child has the ability to …; this is better than trying to guess the power. Also mention what the child is able to do and not able to do. You could always say a neuro-physiotherapy assessment would be useful.

- Comment on atrophy of muscle groups.
- Comment on any movement disorder – dystonia, chorea, athetosis, tremor. Make sure that you are familiar with dystonia, but it can be difficult to characterise other movements. If in doubt you should at least say a 'movement disorder'.
- Examining deep tendon reflexes and grading them is essential: either grade from 1 to 4 (4 being clonus) or say they are 'brisk', 'normal', 'decreased', or 'could not elicit'.
  - Again, inform the parent and the child about what you are about to do and while you are doing it. Many children may have an exaggerated startle and may get upset, which might upset the parent, so anticipate this and give reassurance. It is a good idea to show the child what you will be doing by demonstrating deep tendon reflexes on the parent.
  - Hold the tendon hammer from the base of the handle, and use a good swing to elicit a proper 'stretch reflex'.
  - With proper technique, this should be done only once or twice. If you cannot elicit the reflex, do not persist at the cost of upsetting the child and losing valuable time.
  - Use a blunt object to elicit the plantar response, and say whether it is upgoing (Babinski positive), downgoing, or equivocal.

What scars might you see?

- Look for scars on the hips or upper thighs – femoral osteotomies for hip dislocation.
- Look for scars over the Achilles tendon or on the feet and hands – tendon transfer surgeries.
- Scars on the back – related to scoliosis surgery, or lower back scars are usually due to selective dorsal rhizotomy.

How to summarise your findings

Example: 'My findings on examination are a nine-year-old girl who has a diplegic gait. She wears bilateral rigid ankle–foot orthoses and walks short distances independently. She has increased tone in her lower limbs, and weakness predominantly in the proximal muscle groups of her legs. Her deep tendon reflexes are brisk symmetrically in the lower limbs. My clinical diagnosis is a diplegic cerebral palsy.'

Questions to prepare

- Why are the lower limbs more affected in diplegic cerebral palsy?
- What is meant by cortical visual impairment?
- What is the differential diagnosis of a cerebral palsy-like condition?
- What are the commonest causes of cerebral palsy?
- What are the complications and associated problems of cerebral palsy?
- What are the management approaches and options in cerebral palsy?
- What are the grading systems for cerebral palsy?
- How would you investigate a young child with possible cerebral palsy?

Possible scenarios

- 'Please perform a focused neurological examination on this nine-year-old girl who has some motor difficulties. She was born at term and required no resuscitation at birth. She had global delay in all her milestones and bilateral cataracts. She has limited communication skills and is accompanied by her mother.'
- 'Please perform a focused neurological examination on this five-year-old girl with significant motor difficulties. She was born at term and sustained severe hypoxic–ischaemic encephalopathy. She has global developmental delay and limited communication skills and is accompanied by her mother.'

Chapter 10 **Cranial nerve and ocular examination**

Richard E. Appleton

In paediatric MRCPCH, if cranial nerve examination is required as a specific examination, this will be requested in the 'Neurology' or 'Other' clinical station. If the cranial nerves are examined in MRCPCH, you will usually be asked to examine eye movements (cranial nerves 3, 4, and 6), the face (cranial nerve 7), and the tongue (cranial nerve 12) – which means that you should ensure you can examine these cranial nerves and be able to discuss their most likely anatomical localisation and cause of any abnormalities you find! It is unlikely that you would be asked to examine the other cranial nerves – other than fundoscopy.

From the end of the bed

When you enter the room, greet and talk to the child – as well as their parent – as this may give you important clues. Look at the child's face, eyes, and ears (e.g. the presence of hearing aids); ask the child his or her name, and watch and listen when they respond – as this may reveal dysarthria, dysphasia, facial asymmetry, or some hearing impairment (the child may turn to the parent and sign to them – 'what did he/she say?' – don't miss this rather important clue!).

Clinical Examination Skills in Paediatrics: For MRCPCH Candidates and Other Practitioners, First Edition. Edited by A. Mark Dalzell and Ian Sinha.
© 2020 John Wiley & Sons Ltd. Published 2020 by John Wiley & Sons Ltd.
Companion website: www.wiley.com/go/dalzell/paediatrics

The Following Should Provide you with all you Need to Know about Examination of the Cranial Nerves

Cranial nerve examination

- *1 (Olfactory).* It is very unlikely that this nerve would be formally examined in the clinical examination. Impaired smell will also always involve impaired taste (see also *7 (Facial nerve)*).
- *2 (Optic).* This can be assessed by examining the peripheral visual fields and also the pupillary light response. Absence of a pupillary response (direct and consensual) indicates bilateral optic nerve dysfunction. A lesion of one optic nerve will result in a 'relative afferent pupillary defect'. This means that the pupil of the affected eye will not constrict when a bright light is moved or swung from the normal eye to the affected eye. Fundoscopy is also part of the assessment of the optic nerve. On the rare occasion that the examiner will ask a candidate to examine a child's fundi this will be in a cooperative child and the abnormality is likely to be obvious; specifically: optic atrophy (note that there is always a degree of relative temporal pallor in 'normal' individuals), optic nerve hypoplasia (a very small optic disc), an abnormality of the optic disc (such as a phakoma or coloboma), retinitis pigmentosa, or retinal haemorrhages. It is very unlikely that you will be asked to examine the fundi in a child with papilloedema – although, obviously, you must be able to recognise this important sign (earliest evidence is loss of venous pulsation, then blurring of disc margins, followed by haemorrhages and exudates). Detailed assessments of the visual fields and pupillary responses are addressed at the end of this section.
- *3 (Oculomotor), 4 (Trochlear), and 6 (Abducens).* It is important to assess eye movements (smooth saccades and nystagmus) and to be able to identify a squint; failure to accurately assess and identify a squint will, almost certainly, result in at

least a 'clear fail' in most situations. The cover test is important in identifying a non-paralytic squint. In a non-paralytic squint the squinting eye will be obvious when both eyes are open. When the good, non-squinting eye is covered, the squinting eye will then move, so that it will take up fixation. When the normal eye is then uncovered, the squinting eye will revert to its squinting position. Clearly, if the squint has been present for a number of years, the squinting eye will not be able to do this. If there is thought to be a weakness or paralysis of one or more ocular muscles, the child must be asked to look in six directions – along the lines of the 'Union flag' pattern. When looking for nystagmus on lateral gaze, do not abduct the eyes more than 30–35° as this may induce 'normal', physiological nystagmus.

- *5 (Trigeminal).* This involves assessing facial sensation and facial movement (masseter and temporalis muscles) and the corneal reflex. Palpate the masseter and temporalis muscles with the jaw/teeth clenched and then ask the child to open the jaw against resistance; with a unilateral trigeminal weakness, the jaw will deviate to the paralysed side. Always warn the child before testing the corneal reflex – which should be on the lateral corner of the cornea. The reflex will be reduced in children who wear contact lenses. The corneal reflex will be absent on the affected side and older children will usually be able to describe the difference in the corneal sensation between the two sides.

- *7 (Facial).* The most obvious examination point will be to identify facial asymmetry and facial palsy (it is crucial to be able to demonstrate how to examine the facial nerve and differentiate a lower from an upper motor neurone lesion). Examination of the child's face at rest and asking them to smile, frown, and close their eyes tightly will usually reveal the facial palsy and whether it is lower or upper motor neurone in type. If the upper face and forehead are involved this means that it will be a lower motor neurone problem. Formal assessment includes asking the child to smile; frown; open their eyes widely, close them tight shut, and while they are shut trying to open them again; blow out their cheeks; and purse their lips tightly together, and while they are pursed trying to open them again. Taste in the anterior two-thirds of the tongue is supplied by the facial nerve (the posterior third is supplied by the glossopharyngeal [9th] nerve). The usual tastes that are tested are: sweet (sugar/honey), salt, lemon (bitter), and vinegar with the mouth washed out between each taste. It would be extremely unusual for the examiner to ask the candidate to assess taste in the examination. If you were asked (even theoretically) then you would use: a sweet taste (sugar/honey); salt; bitter (lemon).

- *8 (Acoustic/auditory; remember to look at the child's ears for any hearing aids – particularly in the 'Child development' clinical station).* In the rare situation where you might be asked to formally assess a child's hearing in the clinical examination, it is important to know how to be able to differentiate conductive from sensorineural deafness. Therefore, it is important to know the basic tests and the correct frequency of the tuning fork, which is 512 Hz. In *Weber's test*, the 512 Hz tuning fork is placed on the vertex or mid-line on the upper forehead. Normally, the sound is heard equally in both ears. In perceptive (sensorineural) deafness the sound will be heard louder in the intact (normal) ear. In conductive deafness, it will be heard louder in the affected or deaf ear. In *Rinne's test*, the 512 Hz tuning fork is held against the mastoid process and then just in front of the pinna. In normal children and in children with perceptive (sensorineural) deafness, air conduction is better perceived than bone conduction (called 'Rinne positive'). The reverse is true for conductive deafness. It will be very unusual for candidates to be asked to examine vestibular function.
- *9 (Glossopharyngeal).* Isolated lesions of this nerve are rare. Such lesions usually involves additional cranial nerves and, specifically, nerves 10 and 11. A Chiari malformation may lead to unilateral or bilateral depression of the gag reflex.

Assessment of the gag reflex is with a sterile cotton bud pressed into each tonsillar fossa. The nerve also supplies taste fibres to the posterior third of the tongue – but this is difficult to examine in clinical practice and in children. It is likely to elicit a gag reflex!

- *10 (Vagus).* This will involve an assessment of the uvula and posterior pharyngeal wall. The child should be asked to say 'aah'; and the midline of the soft palate should rise centrally. Unilateral vagal nerve palsy causes palatal deviation – to the intact side – and hoarseness and dysphagia. Bilateral vagal nerve palsies lead to complete palatal paralysis with dysarthria and severe dysphagia. The vocal cords are immobile and rest in an intermediate position and produce stridor on deep inspiration.
- *11 (Accessory).* The cranial nerve component of the 11th nerve cannot be separated from the vagus nerve, in terms of its clinical function. However, the spinal component of the 11th nerve can be assessed. Isolated lesions of the spinal accessory nerve are very rare – and result in weakness of the sternomastoid and trapezius. The sternomastoids are assessed by asking the child to turn his or her head to the side and then try to resist your attempt to return the child's head to the mid-line. If the child cannot resist then that demonstrates weakness of the trapezius and sternomastoid on that side. The trapezii are assessed by asking the child to shrug his or her shoulders without and then against resistance.
- *12 (Hypoglossal).* In a unilateral lower motor neurone lesion, there is ipsilateral atrophy with fasciculation and protrusion of the tongue towards the affected (paralysed) side. Bilateral lower motor neurone lesions cause a bulbar palsy, usually in association with other lower brain stem nuclei, resulting in dysarthria and dysphagia. Unilateral upper motor neurone lesions often have little clinical effect, although there may be some deviation to the affected (paralysed) side. Bilateral upper motor neurone lesions result

Chapter 10

in a pseudo-bulbar palsy – with accompanying dysarthria, dysphagia, and emotional lability. The tongue is stiff and moves slowly; palatal movement is poor and both the palatal and jaw jerks are brisk.

Visual field examination

This is an important part of the assessment of the optic nerve (cranial nerve 2). You should sit approximately 1 m in front of the child and the background (behind you and towards which the child is looking) should be white or certainly plain. A red-headed pin (diameter 5–7 mm) should ideally be used. To test the child's left visual field, the child's right eye should be shut and the examiner's left eye should be shut. The peripheral field can be identified by bringing the pin into the four quadrants of the field. The same is repeated for the child's right visual field. If the red-headed pin is used you should ask the child to tell you when the target appears red, and not just when they can see it. If a red-headed pin is not available, then the examiner's wiggling finger can be used instead. For most of the visual field defects encountered in usual clinical practice this will be adequate. The most common visual field defects that a child might have will be:

1 bi-temporal hemianopia: a defect in the temporal part of both visual fields
2 homonymous hemianopia – a defect in the temporal half of one field and the nasal half of the other.

Pupillary examination

This is an important and relatively easy part of the examination of the optic nerve. Note should be made of the colour of the irides (to ensure they are the same colour), whether there are any cataracts, and the shape and size of the pupils. Up to 20% of the population may have a 'normal', physiological difference of 2 mm between the two pupils (called anisocoria). A defect in the shape of the pupil is termed 'coloboma'. The 'swinging torch' test is used to assess the direct and consensual pupillary responses. The child is asked to fix on a distant object. Swing the torch light from one eye to the other; during this you should only look at the eye that is being illuminated. Normally, as the torch is swung from the first to the second eye, the pupil of the second eye briefly starts to dilate (having lost its consensual response) but then constricts immediately as the torch reaches and illuminates it. If there is a lesion in the optic nerve of the second eye, then the pupil of that eye will continue to dilate as the torch shines on it.

Chapter 10

Chapter 11 Examining a child with a neuromuscular disorder (focusing on Duchenne muscular dystrophy)

Stefan Spinty and Anand S. Iyer

Case scenario which may be presented

Please perform a focused neurological examination on this five-year-old boy who has been referred by his GP because of concerns about his motor abilities. He has delayed gross motor milestones and walked independently at 18 months of age. He was born at term and required no resuscitation at birth. He has easy fatiguability, difficulty climbing stairs, and difficulty getting up from the floor. He also has speech and language delay.

Key points to consider while conducting your examination

- Is this a central or peripheral neurological problem?
- Is the child ambulant?
- If not ambulant, then how does he achieve mobility?
- Review of the wheelchair/assisted devices for mobility.
- Observe the social communication skills.

From the end of the bed

- Observe the child's activities and play.
- Any facial dysmorphism, or neurocutaneous stigmata?

Clinical Examination Skills in Paediatrics: For MRCPCH Candidates and Other Practitioners, First Edition. Edited by A. Mark Dalzell and Ian Sinha.
© 2020 John Wiley & Sons Ltd. Published 2020 by John Wiley & Sons Ltd.
Companion website: www.wiley.com/go/dalzell/paediatrics

- Observe the child's speech – is it clear or muddled, strong or low pitch of voice?
- Is the child ambulant? Observe the gait (waddling in muscle diseases, high stepping in nerve diseases).
- If using walking aids or a wheelchair, note the details.
- Wheelchair – look for a finger-triggered switch, truncal and neck support.
- Does the child have a percutaneous gastrostomy (PEG)?
- Does the child have a tracheostomy, supplementary oxygen, or a suction machine?
- Are there any non-invasive ventilation devices?

Detailed assessment

- Look for calf and shoulder hypertrophy (Duchenne muscular dystrophy [DMD]).
- Look for toe walking (DMD).
- Distal muscle wasting (in both muscular dystrophies and neuropathies).
- Pes cavus, hammer toe, foot deformities, and callouses (hereditary sensory–motor neuropathy).
- Cognitively bright with global severe hypotonia (spinal muscular atrophy).
- Contractures visible (predominantly neuropathies).
- Excessive weight gain (non-ambulant DMDs).
- Cushingoid features (steroid therapy in muscular dystrophies).
- Ptosis, strabismus.

Important signs to look for (and not miss)

- Walking on heel and toe (examining distal muscle strength).
- Gower's sign – the manoeuvre is properly done by asking the child to lie supine on the floor and giving a clear instruction to get up as soon as possible when told. A positive sign is considered when the child turns prone and then climbs up his legs.

Chapter 11

- Look for facial weakness (ask the child to smile and close his eyes tightly).
- Ptosis – ask the child to maintain an upward gaze for a minute. Look for worsening ptosis in myasthenia gravis.
- Look for extraocular eye movements and diplopia (myasthenia gravis).
- Focused motor examination of power, tone, and deep tendon reflexes (not essential if you are short of time and your initial clinical impression is a muscular dystrophy; essential if a neuropathy is suspected).
- Focused sensory examination of vibration, joint position sense, and pain – more important in hereditary sensory–motor neuropathy.
- Look for scars of muscle biopsy (usually quadriceps).
- Look for chest wall deformities (bell-shaped chest in spinal muscular atrophy).
- Look for surgery scars (tendon transfer, femoral osteotomies).
- Look for scoliosis and surgical scars for spinal rod insertion, exaggerated lumbar lordosis indicating truncal muscle weakness.

Additional components of the examination of a child with possible neuromuscular problems

- Plot height, weight, and head circumference on a growth chart.
- Carry out a cardiological examination (cardiomyopathy in muscular dystrophies).

How to summarise your findings

Example. 'My findings on examination are a five-year-old boy who walks on his toes and has a positive Gower's sign. He has calf hypertrophy bilaterally. He does not have any facial weakness or limb weakness. Examination of his power shows proximal muscle weakness, which is symmetrical. He also displays speech delay and autistic features.

My clinical diagnosis is a proximal muscular disorder, and the differentials include muscular dystrophies such as Duchenne muscular dystrophy.'

Questions to prepare

- What are the initial investigations if a muscle disorder is suspected?
- Why does the child have speech delay?
- When would the ambulation be lost in DMD?
- What is the initial treatment to avoid loss of ambulation?

Top tips

- Commonest life-limiting inherited muscular dystrophy in the UK.
- Multisystem disease that affects skeletal muscle, cardiac muscle, brain, gut, and bladder.
- X-linked transmission.
- Symptomatic female carriers can present very rarely.
- About 30% of newly diagnosed children either have a spontaneous mutation or their mother is a carrier of the mutation in all or some of the germ cell line (eggs).
- Second most common inherited disease after cystic fibrosis.
- Affects about 1 : 3600–6000 live-born boys.
- Caused by mutations (exon deletions, duplications, or point mutations) in the dystrophin gene, one of the largest genes in humans, which codes for the dystrophin protein.
- Dystrophin is expressed in skeletal, cardiac, and smooth muscle (bowel, bladder) as well as in brain and other tissues.
- Absent or severely depleted dystrophin leads to a loss of integrity of the muscle cell with subsequent destruction that cannot be overcome by the muscle repair mechanisms.
- Natural history of the disease and its progression are well known.

Chapter 11

- Median predicted survival is currently quoted in the UK as mid- to end twenties.
- Quality of life and life expectancy have improved significantly in recent years with improved surveillance and modern treatment modalities

Presentation

- Most boys with DMD present without a family history because of concerns regarding gross motor developmental delay and associated features.
- A positive family history usually leads to early screening (creatine kinase with subsequent mutation screening via molecular genetics) in the newborn period.
- Some children present with the incidental finding of elevated alanine aminotransferase/aspartate transaminase with normal bilirubin and gamma-glutamyl transferase and no clinical signs of liver disease. Muscle origin is confirmed by estimation of creatine kinase.
- Some present with speech and language delay, learning difficulties, and unusual behaviour but few muscle-related signs or symptoms.
- More recently children are referred with mutations detected via microarray genetic testing done for non-muscle-related reasons (learning difficulties, attention deficit–hyperactivity disorder).

Diagnosis

- Screening via creatine kinase estimation (very high, 100 times the upper limit of normal).
- Raised liver enzymes (muscle derived) and lactate dehydrogenase.
- Diagnosis is confirmed by molecular genetics (multiplex ligation-dependent probe amplification (MLPA) assay, or if negative point mutation screening).
- Muscle biopsy remains the gold standard for diagnosis.
- Genetic counselling should be provided.
- Female carriers are at risk of cardiomyopathy – screening recommended.

Differential diagnosis for grossly elevated creatine kinase

- Other dystrophinopathies: intermediate type or Becker's muscular dystrophy (BMD).
- Limb girdle muscular dystrophies (LGMD).
- Congenital muscular dystrophies (CMD).
- Muscle trauma.
- Burns.
- Myositis.

NB. Always confirm elevated values with a second sample two weeks apart

Clinical features

Early
- Weakness: symmetrical, upper and lower limbs, proximal > distal, fatigue, muscle pain, and cramps in younger age but not as frequently as in BMD.
- Reduced motor function from two to three years, continuous decline.
- Pseudo-hypertrophy of calf and lower arm muscles, at times generalised.
- Gower's sign positive.
- Loss of ambulation at 8–12 years, later if on steroid treatment.

Later
- Joint contractures – especially ankles, also hips, knees, upper limbs/hands.
- Scoliosis.
- Nocturnal hypoventilation, weak cough.
- Cardiomyopathy (dilated).
- Gut dysmotility.
- Death – late teenage/young adulthood secondary to respiratory or cardiac failure; life expectancy significantly improved with respiratory and cardiac support.

Chapter 11

Treatment

- General: review and follow up in the multidisciplinary neuro-muscular clinic.
- Steroids – supervised by specialist team (note that there is a risk of adrenal suppression in long-term steroid treatment).
- Currently researched: oligo nucleotides ('exon skipping') – changing DMD phenotype to BMD phenotype.
- Behaviour problems – advice, psychology support.
- Learning difficulties – assessment and support.
- Constipation – laxatives.
- Contractures – ankle, knee, hip, upper limb: physiotherapy, splinting ankle–foot orthoses, surgical release of Achilles tendon.
- Weight – obesity, later possible weight loss: dietetic advice, gastrostomy, calorie supplements.
- Scoliosis – corrective surgery (spinal rods).
- Swallowing difficulties – modification of food consistency, gastrostomy.
- Respiratory weakness – physiotherapy assessment and support, swimming, incentive spirometry, consider prophylactic or early antibiotics, pneumococcal and influenza vaccination.
- Reduced cough – cough augmentation (breath stacking, cough assist machine).
- Cardiomyopathy – angiotensin-converting enzyme inhibitors, beta-blockers, diuretics.
- Gut dysmotility – laxatives, gastrostomy, rectal wash-outs.
- Life-limiting disease – psychology, advanced care planning including end-of-life planning.

Further reading

Bushby, K., Finkel, R., Birnkrant, D.J. et al. (2010). Diagnosis and management of Duchenne muscular dystrophy, part 1: diagnosis, and pharmacological and psychosocial management. *Lancet Neurol.* 9 (1): 77–93.

Bushby, K., Finkel, R., Birnkrant, D.J. et al. (2010). Diagnosis and management of Duchenne muscular dystrophy, part 2: implementation of multidisciplinary care. *Lancet Neurol.* 9: 177–189.

Muscular Dystrophy Campaign. Home page. www.muscular-dystrophy. org (accessed 12 August 2019).

Chapter 11

Chapter 12 **Musculoskeletal examination**

Liza J. McCann

Key points to consider while conducting your examination

- This station may *not* have a child with a musculoskeletal (MSK) problem; listen carefully to what the examiner is asking you, and focus your examination based on this.
- You may be asked to examine the whole or part of the MSK system, the spine, or a single joint. Joints should be examined using a look, feel, move approach.
- You should be familiar with paediatric Gait Arms Legs Spine (pGALS) and Paediatric Regional Examination of the Musculoskeletal System (pREMS) (assessment guide and videos are available on the Versus Arthritis website (https://www.versusarthritis.org). However, the station is not simply a request to perform pGALS.
- Ask if the child has pain anywhere before you examine; ensure that you do not cause pain.
- Ask about function (dressing, writing, walking up and down stairs easily, tying shoe laces, etc.). Functional tasks can be scored formally by validated questionnaires (Klepper 2003). The Childhood Health Assessment Questionnaire (CHAQ) is used in many paediatric rheumatology units in the UK (see the British Society of Paediatric and Adolescent Rheumatology

Clinical Examination Skills in Paediatrics: For MRCPCH Candidates and Other Practitioners, First Edition. Edited by A. Mark Dalzell and Ian Sinha.
© 2020 John Wiley & Sons Ltd. Published 2020 by John Wiley & Sons Ltd.
Companion website: www.wiley.com/go/dalzell/paediatrics

website [www.bspar.org.uk]; the CHAQ form is available under the 'clinical guidelines' tab).

- Look for clues around the examination couch – check shoes for insoles/pattern of wear and tear, look out for splints, aids, orthotics, crutches, or a wheelchair.
- If asked to examine the lower limbs, asking the child to walk first may provide you with clues as to where to concentrate your examination.
- Practice your MSK examination so that it looks smooth; try to avoid asking the child to keep getting on and off the examination couch – ensure that you have completed all you want to look for while the child is standing/sitting/lying before you ask them to move. Examine gait if possible before the child gets on the couch.
- Think in layers to try to identify where pathology might lie, i.e. skin, fat fascia, tendons, entheses, periosteum, bone, ligaments, synovium, cartilage, articular surfaces, intra-articular structures, effusions.

Possible scenarios

- Scenarios tend to reflect how a child may present in clinic with a complaint (Table 12.1).
- You should be able to recognise the multisystem features associated with arthritis and connective tissue disease and the need to assess other systems as appropriate.
  - For classification and treatment of juvenile idiopathic arthritis (JIA) refer to Espinosa and Gottlieb (2012).
  - For a simple description of classification of childhood scleroderma refer to the Scleroderma Foundation website (http://www.scleroderma.org/site/PageNavigator/patients_whatis.html#.Uch44D771j0).

Examination

General signs to look for
- General well-being: well/unwell; pallor from anaemia.
- Obvious abnormalities of growth, stature, nutritional status/obesity.

Chapter 12

Table 12.1 Possible musculoskeletal (MSK) scenarios in the MRCPCH exam.

Potential scenario	Possible causes (not exhaustive)	Considerations/questions to prepare
This child has difficulty walking. Please examine his/her lower limbs and see if you can suggest a diagnosis. 👁	Arthritis (JIA/septic/reactive). Perthes disease or SUFE. Dermatomyositis (JDM) or polymyositis (JPM). Muscular dystrophy/neurological causes. Contractures due to scleroderma, arthritis, or contracture syndrome. Mechanical joint pains. Haemophilia (with acute or chronic arthritis). Down syndrome (hypertonia and hypermobility with or without arthritis). Rickets. Mucopolysaccharidoses. Malignancies: of bone/haematological/metastatic. Chronic pain syndromes.	May need to perform MSK and neurological examination. Look for dysmorphic features or obvious deformities. Look for muscle wasting/skin rashes/scars/lipoatrophy (generalised or at the site of joint injections) or calcinosis. Check for scoliosis/leg length discrepancy. Consider how to diagnose arthritis by the presence of tenderness, warmth, swelling, or loss of movement and how to differentiate JIA from septic arthritis. Know the subgroups of JIA, consider further investigations (including ophthalmology referral for JIA) and treatment. Growth chart.

| This child has recently developed joint pains and a rash. Can you examine and see if you can suggest a cause. | Arthritis (psoriatic or systemic-onset JIA).
HSP or other vasculitis.
JDM.
JSLE.
Crohn disease with erythema nodosum.
Lyme disease.
Idiopathic urticaria.
Reactive arthritis, e.g. post-streptococcal/ rheumatic fever, viral illness.
Malignancy. | Psoriatic arthritis may affect DIP joints (unusual in other subtypes).
Check for enthesitis.
Look for skin signs of JDM/JSLE. Consider checking muscle strength.
Systemic JIA, vasculitides, JSLE, malignancies may be associated with lymphadenopathy; hepatosplenomegaly, serositis, and other multisystem signs so mention the need for a good general examination including blood pressure and urinalysis.
Further investigations, including urine dipstick and blood pressure for HSP/SLE.
Disease treatment.
Growth chart. |

(*Continued*)

Table 12.1 (Continued)

Potential scenario	Possible causes (not exhaustive)	Considerations/questions to prepare
This child has had swelling/pain/abnormal appearance affecting their legs/hands/back/specific joint. Please examine.	Arthritis JIA. Mechanical joint pains. Perthes. SUFE, DDH. JDM. SLE. Vasculitis. Crohn's/UC. Skeletal dysplasia. Congenital abnormalities, e.g. Poland syndrome. CRMO/SAPHO. Contracture syndromes including arthrogryposis.	Look for dysmorphic features (suggestive of skeletal dysplasia or chromosomal abnormality). Look for skin signs. CRMO/SAPHO can cause clavicle swelling. Look for enthesitis. Look for contractures/asymmetry.
The mother of this child has noticed that he/she is clumsy. Please examine and suggest a possible cause.	BJHS, EDS, Marfan syndrome. Osteogenesis imperfecta. Neurological causes.	Beighton score. Check function (writing). Look for all features of syndromes associated with hypermobility. Check for muscle weakness and say you would do a complete neurological examination.

This child has been complaining of stiffness in her hip. Please examine and suggest possible causes.	Arthritis – including ERA. Crohn disease. Hip pathology: DDH (age 0–3 years), Perthes (age 3–10), SUFE (10–15 years). Secondary osteoarthritis/avascular necrosis post infection or post steroids.	Remember to examine knee if presenting with hip pain (and vice versa). Differentiate hip pathology from SI/spine. Check spinal movement (Schober's), look for tender enthesitis points. Ask about timing of stiffness (early morning stiffness/gelling after inactivity suggests possible JIA).
This child has had difficulty writing; please examine their hands.	Arthritis. Hypermobility/EDS/Marfan syndrome. Neurological causes. Contracture syndrome (including arthrogryposis).	Check writing. Look for features associated with hypermobility. Look for rashes/nail-fold capillaries/scars and other clues.

(Continued)

Table 12.1 (Continued)

Potential scenario	Possible causes (not exhaustive)	Considerations/questions to prepare
The mother of this child has noticed a limp. Please examine.	Leg length discrepancy from DDH, Perthes, SUFE, congenital causes or linear scleroderma. Idiopathic scoliosis. Hemiplegia. Functional. Hip/knee/ankle/foot pathology.	Examine gait, leg lengths, and lower limbs. Look for associated signs that may point to a diagnosis. Consider if a neurological examination is required.
This child has been noticed to have a swollen joint and weight loss. Please examine and consider possible causes.	Arthritis. Crohn's/UC. Vasculitis. Septic arthritis. JDM/JSLE.	Look for signs of arthritis/associated conditions. Plot growth.

BJHS = benign joint hypermobility; CRMO = chronic recurrent multifocal osteomyelitis; DDH = developmental dysplasia of the hip; DIP = distal interphalangeal joint; EDS = Ehlers–Danlos syndrome; ERA = enthesitis-related arthritis; HSP = Henoch– Schönlein purpura; JIA = juvenile idiopathic arthritis; JDM = juvenile dermatomyositis; JPM = juvenile polymyositis; JSLE = juvenile systemic lupus erythematosus; SAPHO = synovitis, acne, pustulosis, hyperostosis, osteitis; SI = sacroiliac; SLE = systemic lupus erythematosus; SUFE, slipped upper femoral epiphysis; UC = ulcerative colitis.

- Dysmorphic features.
- Skin rashes; colour of hands – recognition of poor perfusion.
- Facial abnormalities: deformity or wasting (scleroderma en coup de sabre/Parry–Romberg syndrome), malar rash, juvenile dermatomyositis (JDM) (systemic lupus erythematosus [SLE]).
- Eyes (conjunctivitis, cataract, jaundice).
- Muscle bulk and symmetry (global wasting vs specific muscles or groups).
- Difference in hand/foot size or arm/leg length discrepancy (scleroderma or congenital hemiatrophy).
- Obvious lack of movement/contracture of limb (scleroderma/damage from arthritis/contracture syndrome).
- Obvious gait abnormalities/abnormality of foot position/scoliosis.

Additional features that may be seen by the discerning candidate
- Skin signs suggesting an underlying connective tissue disorder/subcutaneous nodules/nail-fold erythema or nail-fold capillary changes.
- ENT: mouth ulcers/nasal ulceration juvenile systemic lupus erythematosus (JSLE/vasculitis); consider asking about genital ulcers if mouth ulcers are present (Behçet disease). Look at the palate: high arched (Marfan syndrome)/ulcerated (SLE). Look for nasal crusting/blood-stained rhinorrhoea/nasal obstruction/nasal septum perforation/saddle nose deformity/stridor/sinusitis (granulomatosis with polyangiitis, GPA).
- Dentition (poor dental hygiene due to juvenile idiopathic arthritis [JIA]/dental abnormalities with Ehlers–Danlos syndrome [EDS]) or limited mouth opening (JIA with temporomandibular joint [TMJ] involvement/systemic sclerosis); gum hypertrophy with drugs such as ciclosporin.
- Lymphoreticular system (SLE, systemic-onset JIA, malignancy, infection).

Chapter 12

- Circulation: absent peripheral pulses with Takayasu vasculitis; blood pressure (SLE/vasculitis), cardiac murmurs (Marfan syndrome).
- Osteitis of chest wall/clavicle swelling in SAPHO (synovitis, acne, pustulosis, hyperostosis, osteitis) syndrome/chronic recurrent multifocal osteomyelitis (CRMO).
- Ask for urinalysis (vasculitis/SLE).

Essential skin signs to look for
- Psoriasis (including checking scalp/umbilicus/elbows).
- Malar rash JSLE/JDM.
- Urticarial rash/erythema/vasculitis.
- Livido reticularis (JDM, JSLE, vasculitis).
- Skin ulceration (JDM, diabetes, infection, vasculitis).
- Petechial rashes/purpura Henoch–Schönlein purpura (HSP).
- Colour changes that may indicate Raynaud syndrome.
- Wide paper-thin scars, velvety skin, and increased skin elasticity indicate EDS).
- Alopecia (JDM, JSLE).
- Nail changes: onycholysis, nail pitting (psoriasis).

Additional features that may be seen by the discerning candidate
- Abnormal nail-fold erythema/dilated capillaries (JDM/scleroderma).
- Heliotrope discoloration of eyelids (JDM).
- Gottron's patches (JDM).
- Calcinosis (JDM or systemic sclerosis).
- Lipoatrophy (JDM, scleroderma, or local lipoatrophy at sites of joint injections in JIA).
- Tight shiny skin, subcutaneous wasting (scleroderma).
- Skin pigmentation (localised scleroderma, JDM).
- Digital pits/ulcers, sclerodactyly (systemic sclerosis).
- Digital infarction (systemic sclerosis).
- Telangiectasia (limited systemic sclerosis).

Chapter 12

For pictures of all the skin signs listed above, refer to the American College Rheumatology image bank (http://images.rheumatology.org); follow the link to Rheumatic Diseases of Childhood for images of JIA, SLE, JDM, scleroderma, and vasculitis. For pictures on hypermobility/EDS/Marfan syndrome/osteogenesis imperfecta, follow the link to Heritable Disorders of Connective Tissue. Images for dermatomyositis can also be found at http://escholarship.org/uc/item/1f04d17z.

Gait examination

- Observe for symmetry, smoothness, and ability to turn quickly.
- Look briefly at the child's head (head bobbing may suggest a limp). Look for symmetry elsewhere (shoulders, hips, legs), obvious muscle wasting, or skin changes.
- Walking pattern: smooth pattern with appropriate arm swing, heel–toe propulsion.
- Look for any foot abnormalities (excessive high arch/low arch, clawing of toes, hallux valgus, foot deformities, pronation).
- Look for spinal alignment, gluteal bulk and symmetry, knee flexion or hyperextension.
- Ask the child to walk on tip-toes. Normal arch?
- Ask the child to walk on their heels (inability due to pain may suggest enthesitis).
- Ask the child to stand on one leg, bend the knee slightly/hop (testing balance, coordination, quadriceps function).

Types of gait
- Antalgic gait due to a painful limb, often resulting in a limp (shortened stance phase with the foot on the ground on the affected side).
- Waddling gait (wide-based) – pelvic muscle girdle weakness; seen in myopathy (e.g. muscular dystrophy/JDM).
- Trendelenburg (pelvis tilts downwards on the weakened affected side during stance phase) from muscle weakness or hip pathology.

Chapter 12

- Steppage gait (difficulty clearing toes during the swing phase due to foot drop; may be associated with vasculitis).
- Toe walking (avoiding putting weight on the heel); may be habitual but can be associated with neurological disease/gastrocnemius contracture/JIA.
- Circumduction gait – circular movement of the leg with excessive hip abduction as the leg swings forward (leg length discrepancy/lack of full knee extension/hemiplegic cerebral palsy).
- Abnormal gait due to neurological impairment: hemiplegia/spastic diplegia, cerebellar ataxia.

Examination of arms
- General: muscle bulk, asymmetry, contractures, deformity, swollen joints, rashes, nail changes, scars, skin elasticity.

Hands and wrists
- Look: for swelling (synovitis/dactylitis), rashes (psoriasis, palmar erythema, pigmentation changes), symmetry, deformity, muscle wasting, scars, skin thinning or bruising (possibly indicating long-term steroid use), arachnodactyly (Marfan syndrome), deformities, or contractures.
- Feel: for warmth, tenosynovitis, synovitis (palpating individual joints).
- Move: range of movement (active and passive) of all joints of fingers, thumbs, and wrists including checking for hypermobility.
- Function: ability to make a fist; buttons/writing.

Additional features that may be seen by the discerning candidate
- Skin signs suggestive of JDM/scleroderma: Gottron's patches, nail-fold changes, sclerodactyly/digital pits/nodules.
- Detailed description of deformities: swan neck deformities, Z-thumb (hyperextension of the interphalangeal joint and fixed flexion/subluxation of the metacarpophalangeal joint), Boutonniere's deformity, Dupuytren's contracture.

- Consider checking peripheral pulses (may be absent in Takayasu vasculitis).
- Consider testing median, ulnar, and radial nerve power.
- Assess power and grip strength.

Elbows
- Look: for carrying angle, scars, contractures, swelling, rashes (such as psoriasis).
- Feel: skin temperature, synovitis, tendonitis (palpate joint).
- Move: range of movement (active and passive) – flexion, extension, pronation, supination, note any hyperextension.
- Function: moving hand to nose or mouth/behind head.

Shoulder
- Look: fullness/muscle wasting, angulation, misalignment, clavicle swelling.
- Feel: skin temperature, palpation of bony landmarks for tenderness (tendonitis/bursitis/arthritis).
- Move: range of movement (active and passive) – flexion, extension, abduction, adduction, external rotation, internal rotation.

Examination of legs – general tests
Leg length
Align the pelvis and measure from the anterior superior iliac spine to the medial malleolus of the same leg.

Trendelenburg test
Ask the child to lift one leg and watch for a tilt of the pelvis on the non-weight-bearing side. Positive test: when the pelvis tilts downwards instead of raising on the side of the lifted foot (indicating weakness on the contralateral stance leg due to conditions such as dislocation of the hip, abductor weakness, or shortening of the femoral neck).

Gower's sign
From supine, ask the child to roll prone (salient feature; normal in toddlers but rarely seen after the age of three years in healthy

Chapter 12

children), extending arms and legs far apart. With most weight on the extended arms, the child pushes their body backwards. Early changes of muscle weakness include exaggerated torso flexion, wide base, and equinus posturing. To extend the hip, the child places hands onto their knees and 'walks' their arms up the thighs until upright (only seen when muscle weakness becomes more pronounced). A child 'rolling prone to rise' but without the full walking up the thighs is still significant. Free online supplementary video material is available demonstrating Gower's sign in four patients with different degrees of weakness (Chang et al. 2012).

Hip
- Look: for flexion deformity, leg length discrepancy, scars, gluteal muscle bulk.
- Feel: for tenderness around greater trochanter.
- Move: range of movement of hip (active and passive) – flexion, extension, internal and external rotation, abduction and adduction. (Inflammatory hip disease and slipped upper femoral epiphysis [SUFE] tend to cause restriction in internal rotation associated with groin pain; mechanical pain tends to cause pain on the lateral side of the hip.) Check straight leg raise. When standing, assess Trendelenburg and gait. Examine knee for possibility of referred pain.
- Function: check gait, particularly looking for an antalgic/Trendelenburg gait, and Gower's sign.

Straight leg raise
Ask the child to lift the leg straight and dorsiflex the foot. It is a positive test if this causes pain in the lower back/leg. Also allows testing of hamstring tightness.

Additional features that may be seen by the discerning candidate
- Thomas's test: to assess occult hip flexion. Place one hand under the child's back to ensure normal lumbar lordosis is removed. Flex the child's knee on one side and push it against the abdomen so that the hip is fully flexed. If the opposite leg

lifts off the couch, it suggests that a fixed flexion deformity is present.
- Pain on sacroiliac stretching suggesting enthesitis – Faber test: place one foot on the opposite knee just above the patella (to flex, abduct, and externally rotate the hip). Press the flexed knee and opposite anterior superior sacroiliac crest down into the examination couch. Pain in the groin indicates a problem in the hip, whereas tenderness in the opposite sacroiliac area indicates a problem in the sacroiliac joints. Repeat on the other side.

Knee
- Look: from the end of the bed for swelling, misalignment (varus deformity, bow legged; valgus deformity, knock kneed), scars, muscle wasting (particularly quadriceps). Look from the side for fixed flexion deformity/scars.
- Feel: skin temperature, palpate the joint line (with knee slightly flexed). Feel the popliteal fossa (check for a popliteal cyst). Patella tap and bulge test to check for effusion. Feel for crepitus while moving the knee.
- Move: assess the range of movement (active and passive) – flexion, extension. Consider checking for hamstring/quadriceps tightness. Examine the hip for the possibility of referred pain.
- Function: consider checking muscle strength. Check gait and balance.

Patellar tap
With the knee extended, squeeze fluid from the suprapatellar pouch and push the patella down with the other hand.

Bulge test
With the knee extended, massage the medial aspect of the knee joint upwards to empty the medial compartment of fluid, then stroke that lateral side downwards distally while looking for a bulge in the medial compartment of the knee indicating an effusion.

Chapter 12

Additional features that may be seen by the discerning candidate
- With the knee flexed, look for tibial tuberosity prominence and feel for tibial tuberosity tenderness (Osgood–Schlatter disease).
- Clarke's test: fix the patella between your fingers and thumb (with the knee extended but relaxed) and ask the child to push their leg down into the bed as hard as they can. You will feel the quadriceps muscle tighten. Pain (if it is the same pain that they are complaining of) suggests anterior knee pain.
- Stability testing (if history of clunking/instability):
  - Varus stress – testing the contralateral ligament. Slightly flex the knee, place one hand on the opposite side of the joint line to the side that you are testing and alternately stress the joint line on each side. Watch for degree of motion and check for discomfort. (Refer to Versus Arthritis handbook and DVDs for more details.)
  - Anterior and positive draw test: with the hip and knee flexed and the foot flat on the examination couch, place your hands on the child's lower leg with your thumbs on the tibia and fingers on the calf muscle while stabilising the lower tibia with your forearm. Pull anteriorly and posteriorly to assess for laxity of the cruciate ligaments (movement beyond 5 mm is considered positive although in young children this degree of movement may be normal).
  - McMurray test for meniscal injury: flex the child's hip and knee to 90° with the foot flat on the examination couch. Hold the heel with the right hand, steady the knee with your thumb and index finger of your left hand on either side of the joint. Extend the knee slowly with the right hand, while palpating the joint line with the left hand. Repeat with the tibia in external and internal rotation (positive test when a clunk is felt with associated pain).

Foot and ankle
- Look: for swelling, scars, deformity, misalignment.
- Feel: skin temperature, joint lining of ankle joints, subtalar and mid-feet.

- Move: assess the range of movement (active and passive) of the ankle (dorsi- and plantarflexion), subtalar (inversion and eversion), mid-tarsal joints (passive rotation), and toes (dorsi- and plantarflexion).
- Function: assess gait. Look at footwear.

Additional features that may be seen by the discerning candidate
- Consider checking peripheral pulses (especially if there are signs of vasculitis).
- Feel for tenderness over enthesitis points on the foot.

Spine
- Look: inspect from the side and from behind. Check for scoliosis, lordosis, or kyphosis.
- Feel: spinal processes, paraspinal muscles.
- Move: lumbar flexion, extension, lateral flexion and rotation of lumbar and cervical spine (ensure sitting up straight or standing when assessing cervical extension; if slouching, extension will appear to be falsely limited).
- Measure: check for leg length discrepancy.
- Function: check gait.

Additional features that may be seen by the discerning candidate
- Palpate sacroiliac dimples for pain/discomfort.
- When lying on the couch, check for hamstring tightness (falsely limiting spinal flexion), straight leg raise and reflexes.
- Consider checking sensation, tone, power.
- Carry out Schober's test if limited lumbar spine mobility is suspected.

Schober's test
Put a pen mark in the midline at the level of the sacroiliac dimples. Place another mark 10 cm above this. Ask the child to bend forward as far as they can, keeping their legs straight. Measure the distance between the pen marks while the child is flexed; should

Chapter 12

increase from 10 cm to 15 cm. Limitation may be due to spinal pathology (such as enthesitis-related arthritis) or tight hamstrings.

Temporomandibular joints
- Look for micrognathia (underdeveloped lower jaw and retracted chin).
- Feel: for tenderness around the TMJ joint.
- Move: ask the child to open and close the jaw, move the lower jaw (chin) backwards and forwards and from side to side. Can they get three fingers (their index middle and ring finger side to side between upper and lower teeth) in their mouth?

Examining for hypermobility
Beighton score
- Passive apposition of the whole thumb to the flexor side of the forearm on both sides (2 points).
- Passive dorsiflexion of the fifth finger metacarpophalangeal joint $\geq 90°$ on both sides (2 points).
- Passive hyperextension of the elbow to $\geq 10°$ on both sides (2 points).
- Passive hyperextension of the knee to $\geq 10°$ on both sides (2 points).
- Palms of hands resting easily on the floor when the spine flexed and legs are straight (1 point).

Additional features that may be seen by the discerning candidate:
- Check for hypermobility in other joints not included in the Beighton score but commonly hypermobile in children: cervical spine extension, shoulders, hips, feet/ankles ('kissing feet' sign: soles of feet touching when feet inverted while the child is supine).
- Look for other signs that may indicate an associated condition (Marfan syndrome/EDS/osteogenesis imperfecta):
  - Skin elasticity/translucency. Striae. Dystrophic, wide, paper-thin scars. Easy bruising.
  - Blue sclera. Lens dislocation or myopia (ophthalmology review).

- High arched palate. Abnormal dentition (dental crowding due to narrow and high arched palate/periodontitis/enamel abnormalities).
- Arachnodactyly.
- Arm span > height.
- Chest wall deformities (pectus excavatum/carinatum).
- Cardiac murmurs.
- Scoliosis/thoracolumbar kyphosis.
- Foot deformity/pes planus.
- Wrist sign – positive when the tip of the thumb covers the entire fingernail of the 5th finger when wrapped around the contralateral wrist.
- Thumb sign –adducting thumb across hand with fingers flexed; positive when entire distal phalanx of the adducted thumb extends beyond the ulnar border of the palm.

Acknowledgements

Thank you to the patients and paediatric rheumatology colleagues at Alder Hey Hospital, Liverpool, and Newcastle Hospital NHS Foundation Trust/Newcastle University for their comments and suggestions.

References

Chang, R.F. and Mubarak, S.J. (2012). Pathomechanics of Gowers' sign: a video analysis of a spectrum of Gowers' maneuvers. *Clin. Orthop. Relat. Res.* 470: 1987–1991.

Espinosa, M. and Gottlieb, B.S. (2012). Juvenile idiopathic arthritis. *Pediatr. Rev.* 33 (7): 303–313.

Klepper, S.E. (2003). Measures of pediatric function. The Childhood Health Assessment Questionnaire (CHAQ), Juvenile Arthritis Functional Assessment Report (JAFAR), Juvenile Arthritis Functional Assessment Scale (JAFAS), Juvenile Arthritis Functional Status Index (JASI) and Pediatric Orthopedic Surgeons of North America (POSNA) pediatric musculoskeletal functional health questionnaire. Arthritis. *Rheum.* 49 (5S): S5–S14.

Chapter 12

Chapter 13 **Examining a child with endocrine problems**

Poonam Dharmaraj, Urmi Das and
Renuka Ramakrishnan

Approach to the examination of a child with short stature

- Before you start examining the child it is important to remember that a child with short stature can be perfectly healthy, as in cases of familial short stature or constitutional delay in growth and puberty.
- Any chronic disease, for example coeliac disease or inflammatory bowel disease, may present with short stature.
- Children with Ullrich–Turner syndrome, Russell–Silver syndrome, Prader–Willi syndrome, and Noonan syndrome present with short stature but there are specific features of each syndrome which will help you make the diagnosis.
- Obvious skeletal dysplasias such as achondroplasia are not difficult to identify but hypochondroplasia may be quite difficult.

Keeping all of the above in mind before you start your examination request the following as appropriate.

- Birth weight and gestational age.
- Growth chart to plot current height and weight.
- Parents' heights to plot the mid-parental target and range.

Clinical Examination Skills in Paediatrics: For MRCPCH Candidates and Other Practitioners, First Edition. Edited by A. Mark Dalzell and Ian Sinha.
© 2020 John Wiley & Sons Ltd. Published 2020 by John Wiley & Sons Ltd.
Companion website: www.wiley.com/go/dalzell/paediatrics

- Sitting height. This can be plotted on a sitting height chart and when subtracted from the total height gives the sub-ischial leg length, which can also be plotted. The ratio between these two (sitting height and sub-ischial leg length) gives clues to a skeletal dysplasia.
- If you know the child was born prematurely request a growth chart specific for gestational age and you will be able to see if the child was born small for gestational age (SGA).
- Bone age.
- In familial short stature bone age is equal to chronological age and the child's height will be within the mid-parental range with normal growth velocity.
- In constitutional delay in growth and puberty, growth velocity may be normal but bone age is delayed.
- SGA is defined as birth weight/length at least two standard deviations below the mean for gestational age; 90% of children born SGA demonstrate 'catch up' growth by two years of age but 10% are still small for their age and may benefit from growth hormone therapy.
- Children with skeletal dysplasias such as achondroplasia present with rhizomelic shortening of their limbs (shortening of the humerus and femur), a large head (can have hydrocephalus), and bow legs with a waddling gait.
- A child with hypochondroplasia may have subtle features that may initially be difficult to diagnose. It is an autosomal dominant condition that presents with disproportionate short stature, with relatively short legs, micromelia, and lumbar lordosis. A sitting height will be helpful to point towards skeletal dysplasia.
- As part of your examination look for signs of any chronic disease such as clubbing, mouth ulcers, cyanosis.
- A girl with Turner syndrome will present with short stature and will possibly be on growth hormone. Don't forget to ask about hearing, renal, and autoimmune problems.
- Pubertal induction with oestrogen is usually done around 12–13 years of age.
- For examination of a child with Prader–Willi syndrome.

Examination of a swelling in the neck

- Equipment needed: stethoscope, glass of water.
- When asking permission to examine the child, note their voice (hoarseness can occur in older children with hypothyroidism).

Signs from the end of the bed
Hyperthyroidism
- Restlessness.
- Exophthalmos.
- Tremor.

Hypothyroidism
- Short stature.
- Thyroidectomy scar.

General points
- Goitre may be present in either hyper- or hypothyroidism.
- Ask to see the growth chart.
- Always have the child seated on a chair if possible for neck examination.
- Inspect for:
  - redness
  - swelling – size/shape/symmetry.
- Confirm it is the thyroid with a glass of water – should move on swallowing.
- Neck palpation – always from behind.
- Ask the child to lower their chin and slightly incline their head towards whichever side is being examined (relaxes overlying sternomastoid).
- Describe:
  - size, shape, symmetry
  - surface, consistency, mobility
  - hot or tender?
- Palpate lobes for a thrill.

- Check the trachea is not displaced.
- Check for draining lymph nodes.
- Percuss across the upper sternum for retrosternal extension of a goitre (will be dull).
- Auscultate over the gland for a bruit.
- If exophthalmos is present or if you are asked to assess the child's eyes as part of a thyroid examination:
  - look from behind over the child's forehead for proptosis
  - look from the side for the same
  - assess lid retraction from the front
  - assess lid lag from the front using your finger – ask the child to track it in a vertical line downwards
  - assess for squint (ophthalmoplegia), extraocular movements (muscle paresis in exophthalmos), and visual fields (mid-line tumour causing hypothyroidism).

Important signs to look for (and not miss)

- Skin – hot/cold, doughy (hypothyroidism), sweaty (hyperthyroidism), flushed, vitiligo (autoimmune).
- Pretibial myxoedema – dorsal aspect feet/legs (hyperthyroidism).
- Hair – dry (hypothyroidism), greasy (hyperthyroidism), alopecia (autoimmune).
- Ask the child to hold out their arms with fingers outstretched – tremor? (hyperthyroidism).
- Pulse.
- Reflexes – brisk (hyperthyroidism), delayed relaxation (hypothyroidism).
- Power (proximal myopathy in hypothyroidism or hyperthyroidism).

Examination of a child with suspected primary adrenal insufficiency (Addison disease)

Possible causes include an autoimmune process affecting only the adrenals or part of polyglandular disease, due to congenital adrenal hyper/hypoplasia, infections like HIV/tuberculosis, metabolic diseases such as Smith–Lemli–Opitz syndrome, in adrenoleukodystrophy, metastatic cancer, etc.

- Plot height and weight (looking for poor growth and weight loss).
- Hair – look for alopecia.
- Skin – look for vitiligo, candidiasis, hyperpigmentation especially in moles, scars, palmar creases, axillae.
- Nails – look for dystrophy.
- Oral cavity – look for hyperpigmentation of lips, gums, oral mucosa, candidiasis.
- Neck – look for goitre (for associated autoimmune disorders).
- Measure blood pressure lying down and standing (can have orthostatic hypotension).
- Other features include possible lack of axillary/pubic hair, poor pubertal progress, prone to develop hypocalcaemia if the child has associated hypoparathyroidism.
- Look for MedicAlert bracelets/chains.
- Assess for any developmental delay.

Examination of a child with suspected steroid excess (Cushing syndrome and Cushing disease)

Possible causes include iatrogenic steroids, adrenal tumour (isolated or as part of tumour syndromes), McCune–Albright syndrome, adrenocorticotropic hormone (ACTH)-secreting pituitary tumour etc.

- Plot height and weight (looking for short stature and obesity).
- The child will have central obesity with a supraclavicular pad of fat.
- Face – look for 'moon face', plethora, acne, hirsutism.
- Examine fundi and field (looking for papilloedema, bitemporal hemianopia).

- Skin – look for violaceous striae, bruising, or ecchymosis (due to skin thinning), acanthosis, hyperpigmentation (ACTH-producing tumours), lanugo hair.
- Back – look for kyphosis, spinal tenderness (due to osteoporosis).
- Check blood pressure.
- Look for proximal muscle weakness.
- Pubertal assessment (can have poor pubertal progress).

Chapter 14 Examining a child with diabetes

Mark Deakin

Key points to consider while conducting your examination

From the end of the bed

- Appearance – does the child look well/unwell?
- Is the child alert or not?
- Does the child seem either underweight or overweight?
- Is there any evidence of thyroid dysfunction (goitre/dry skin/ facies, etc.)?
- Acanthosis nigricans is a non-specific brown–black skin discoloration seen in several endocrine disorders; these include diabetes, hypothyroidism, and Addison disease. In diabetes it is caused by insulin resistance and is most commonly found (in type 2 diabetes) as discoloration on the neck and axillae

Important signs to look for (and not miss)

- Although children attending the examination are unlikely to be acutely ill, it is important that you understand about fluid status. Assessment of cardiovascular status gives a lot of information about fluid balance; high blood glucose causes an osmotic diuresis and volume depletion. Children compensate (using Starling's law) by raising their stroke volume and rate. A difference between central and peripheral capillary refill time shows that peripheral vasoconstriction is being

Clinical Examination Skills in Paediatrics: For MRCPCH Candidates and Other Practitioners, First Edition. Edited by A. Mark Dalzell and Ian Sinha.
© 2020 John Wiley & Sons Ltd. Published 2020 by John Wiley & Sons Ltd.
Companion website: www.wiley.com/go/dalzell/paediatrics

used to maintain central organ perfusion. Skin turgor is a cruder measure of this.

- Respiratory signs are usually uncommon in children with diabetes unless they have another medical condition such as cystic fibrosis or asthma. Increased respiratory rate should always be assessed in the context of potential compensation for acidosis caused by hyperglycaemia.
- Gastrointestinal:
  - Visceromegaly: newly diagnosed children with diabetes often have hepatomegaly due to increased glycogen storage. The same can be palpated in children with poor glycaemic control.
- Lipoatrophy: loss of subcutaneous fat from repeated insulin injections.
- Lipohypertrophy: firm lumps of subcutaneous tissue because of hypertrophy due to repeated insulin injections.
- Long-term hyperglycaemia can cause autonomic dysfunction leading to gastroparesis/slow bowel transit and even urinary retention.
- Oral/urethral thrush can be suggestive of hyperglycaemia.

Nervous system

- Hand/foot sensation: 'stocking and glove' sensory loss is a marker of poor glycaemic control. Classic 'stocking and glove' sensory loss is very rare in children unless they have had poor glycaemic control for many years.
- Hand/foot proprioception: proprioception tends to be preserved longer than sensation, but is another marker of poor glycaemic control.
- Autonomic dysfunction.
- Retinal changes: small 'dot and blot' haemorrhages are a marker of poor glycaemic control; this is termed background retinopathy. These may then progress to haemorrhages and be followed by new vessel growth. As the degree of eye disease increases so does the risk of visual loss. Children over 12 years

of age are enrolled in the retinopathy screening programme and are invited to attend for retinal photography each year.

Examine the injection sites

Most children with diabetes receive between two and five injections per day. The most common injection sites are the lateral aspects of upper arms and thighs, buttocks, and abdomen. The frequency of the injections can lead to 'favourite spots', depending on the handedness of the child and their ability to rotate sites and position within the sites. Areas of lipohypertrophy occur when insulin is repeatedly injected into the same area of skin. Lipoatrophy is rarer and is the localized loss of fat tissue from repeated injection of insulin into the same site. Insulin absorption is reduced in both areas of lipohypertrophy or atrophy.

Additional components of the diabetes examination

Say you would like to examine the urine, and test for proteinuria and glycosuria.

Chapter 15 **Examining a toddler with motor delay**

Melissa Gladstone and Ruairi Gallagher

Key points to consider while conducting your examination

- The size, or perceived age, of the child is unimportant – just because a child looks five years old does not mean he/she has attained the skills of a five-year-old child.
- What is the child doing when you enter the room? This is the baseline for the assessment.
- Never proceed in reverse developmental order – if a child is observed walking do not assess if they can sit unaided or roll over!
- Does the child have any dysmorphic features? Do they have an easily recognisable syndrome (never ignore the 'elephant in the room' – if a child looks like they have trisomy 21 then comment on this when you summarise but tell the examiner you would like to examine the child further to confirm this).
- Remember that this is an examination of motor skills and not a neurological assessment. To some extent, ignore neurological difficulties and assess skill attainment. Neurological difficulties may impact on a child's ability to demonstrate a skill, and this should be noted, but should not be the focus of the examination.

Clinical Examination Skills in Paediatrics: For MRCPCH Candidates and Other Practitioners, First Edition. Edited by A. Mark Dalzell and Ian Sinha.
© 2020 John Wiley & Sons Ltd. Published 2020 by John Wiley & Sons Ltd.
Companion website: www.wiley.com/go/dalzell/paediatrics

- When you enter the room:
  - Listen to the examiner's instructions. They may give you a clue as to the cause of any motor delay, e.g. 'please examine the motor development of this two-year-old child who was born prematurely and has had heart surgery'.
  - Observe what the child is doing – this will be your starting point.
  - Engage with the child – sit on the floor if you think this will help with rapport.

Examination points

- Your aim should be to get the child to perform the skills in advancing developmental order, e.g. if the child is sitting unsupported then aim for the following, in advancing developmental order:

Pull to stand	Coasting	Walking	Running	Jumping

- If the child does not perform a skill, this could mean either that:
  - he/she will not perform it, or
  - he/she has not attained that skill yet.
  In either case, you should ask the parent/carer.
- If the child cannot perform the next skill in a series, then you have identified the current developmental level (the most advanced skill achieved by the child). You should use your knowledge of developmental attainment to guide you to an appropriate developmental level.
- If the child, according to the parent, can perform the next skill, then continue to question the parent regarding the advancing developmental skills until you reach a ceiling (the skill the child cannot perform). Again, when you have identified the last achieved skill in an advancing series, the developmental level of the child has been identified.

Interpretation

- The developmental level (which corresponds to a developmental age) of a child is then compared with the chronological age of the child (e.g. approximate gross motor developmental age of two years at a chronological age of three years).
- The child is either developmentally delayed or age appropriate (even if their skills are advanced!).
- If the child has delay in all four domains of development (gross motor, fine motor/vision, speech and language, and social) they can be described as having 'global developmental delay'. If they have delay in one or two domains then it is 'specific' developmental delay.

How to summarise your findings

'From my examination, I have found that _____

- has age-appropriate motor skill/delayed development of motor skills.
- The evidence for this is that the child has achieved the skill of _____ but cannot yet _____.
- He/she has evidence of dysmorphic features that may be in keeping with a diagnosis of/syndrome (namely, _____), which may explain the motor delay.
- This child has had a history of _____, which may explain the motor delay.
- This child will need developmental support for their motor delay (in the form of physiotherapy/occupational therapy, etc.) and may need further investigation.'

Questions to prepare

- What do you think about the rest of this child's development? (Although you have not formally examined the other domains, be prepared to answer this question. For example, what were the child's fine motor skills and language like?)

- Are there other examinations you would like to perform? (For example, other aspects of development, neurology if possibly hypo/hypertonic, cardiovascular syndrome if cyanosed, etc.)
- What do you think this child's cause of delay is?
- What are the causes of motor delay?
- Who should be involved in the care of this child?
- What investigations might you wish to undertake?

Top tips

- If you are having trouble engaging a child then use the parent to your advantage. Ask them to get the child to do the skill or get them involved (e.g. by getting everyone in the room jumping so you can see the child jumping).
- Do not spend too long trying to engage a child or getting him or her to perform a particular skill. You may run out of time.
- Do not ask a child to do something that is much too advanced. This may not be safe and you will risk the child becoming disengaged.
- Do not take a history of previous development – it is not a history-taking station.
- Do not be worried about saying that a child has delayed development in the presence of a parent. They know why they are there and will be aware of the delay.

Chapter 16 **Examining a toddler with speech delay**

Ruairi Gallagher and Melissa Gladstone

Key points to consider while conducting your examination

- The size, or perceived age, of the child is unimportant – just because a child looks five years old does not mean he/she speaks and understands like an average five-year-old child.
- Pay close attention to everything a child says. You could easily miss something which helps in defining their developmental level/age.
- In assessing speech and language you are also assessing understanding, which has implications for other aspects of the child's development and care.
- Is there a reason for any speech difficulties, e.g. trisomy 21, autism (see Chapter 17), evidence of operations (lip and palate repair, tracheostomy scar)?
- When you enter the room:
  - Listen to the instructions. They may give you a clue as to the cause of any speech delay, e.g. 'please examine the speech development of this two-year-old child who was born prematurely'.
  - Introduce yourself, wash your hands, and state to the parent/carer and child what the purpose of your examination will be and how you will do it.

Clinical Examination Skills in Paediatrics: For MRCPCH Candidates and Other Practitioners, First Edition. Edited by A. Mark Dalzell and Ian Sinha.
© 2020 John Wiley & Sons Ltd. Published 2020 by John Wiley & Sons Ltd.
Companion website: www.wiley.com/go/dalzell/paediatrics

- Observe what the child is saying and doing – this will be your starting point.
- Engage with the child – sit on the floor if the child is also on the floor and if you think this will help with rapport.

Important signs to look for (and not miss)

- Your aim in developmental assessment should generally be to get the child to perform the skills in advancing developmental order. However, in speech assessment this is more challenging and more attention will need to be paid to the natural conversation. For example, the child may, spontaneously, say a six-word sentence with information contained within the sentence that aids in your assessment.
- If the child does not talk, this could mean either:
  - that he/she will not talk to you, or
  - he/she has not attained that skill yet.
  - In either case, you should ask the parent/carer. This also applies to a case where you attempt to get a child to tell you something (e.g. colours) and they do not or cannot. If in doubt, ask the parent.
- The developmental level/age attained corresponds to the most advanced speech and language demonstrated by the child and/or that which the parent informs you.

Interpretation

- The developmental level (which corresponds to a developmental age) of a child is then compared with the chronological age of the child.
- The child is either developmentally delayed or age appropriate (even if their speech skills are advanced!).
- A child is likely to have specific speech delay if their understanding is age appropriate and expressive speech is delayed. If both are delayed, they are likely to have global developmental delay.

How to summarise your findings

'From my examination, I have found that _____

- has age-appropriate speech/delayed development of speech skills.
- The evidence for this is that this child can _____ but cannot _____.
- Although I have not examined this child specifically, he/she has evidence of dysmorphic features that may be in keeping with a diagnosis of/syndrome namely, _____, which may explain the speech delay.
- This child has had a history of _____, which may explain the speech delay.
- This child will need developmental support for his/her speech delay (in the form of speech and language therapy and educational support) and may need further investigation (e.g. hearing).'

Questions to prepare

- What do you think about the rest of this child's development? (Although you have not formally examined the other domains, be prepared to answer this question. For example, what were the child's motor and social skills like?)
- Are there other examinations you would like to perform (e.g. other aspects of development, neurology, etc.)?
- What do you think the cause of this child's delay is?
- What are the causes of speech delay?
- Who should be involved in the care of this child?
- What investigations might you wish to undertake?
- What did you think of this child's communication/social skills?
- How do you think this child's speech delay impacts on their friendships/play/education?

Top tips

- If you are having trouble engaging a child then use the parent to your advantage. Ask them to get involved in any games, reading a book, or in talking about colours/body parts/counting etc.
- Do not spend too long trying to engage a child. You may run out of time for your examination.
- Do not take a history of previous speech development (e.g. 'When did he first say any words?'). This is irrelevant to the current speech examination.

Chapter 17 **Examining a child with autism**

Ruairi Gallagher and Melissa Gladstone

Key points to consider while conducting your examination

- If asked to examine a child with autism spectrum disorder (ASD), you could either perform a physical examination looking for associations (e.g. fragile X syndrome, tuberous sclerosis) or a developmental assessment (probably assessing speech and language with associated social communication difficulties). If it's a developmental station then, obviously, the latter is required.
- Not all children with ASD have 'classical' autism (autism with moderate/severe learning difficulties).
- Look for evidence of associated comorbidities such as learning difficulties, speech delay, attention deficit hyperactivity disorder (ADHD), co-ordination difficulties.

Important signs to look for (and not miss)

Developmental assessment
- When assessing social communication skills, look for, and comment on, use of eye contact, use of body language and gesture, and use of language. Remember, they may all be present but it is the quality that you are assessing.
- Try to engage the child in imaginative role play.

Clinical Examination Skills in Paediatrics: For MRCPCH Candidates and Other Practitioners, First Edition. Edited by A. Mark Dalzell and Ian Sinha.
© 2020 John Wiley & Sons Ltd. Published 2020 by John Wiley & Sons Ltd.
Companion website: www.wiley.com/go/dalzell/paediatrics

Chapter 17

- Read a picture book together to assess the child's responses to character emotions and meanings of stories and idioms.
- Ask about friendships ('Do you have friends?', 'What does being a best friend mean to you?') and annoyances ('What annoys you?', 'Do you ever annoy other people?'). This will provide some insight into their interpretation of friendships and their insight into their peer relations.

Physical examination

- Measure height, weight, and head circumference.
- Assess cardiovascular, respiratory, gastrointestinal, and neurological systems.
- Examine the patient's skin (use a Wood's lamp if it is available).
- Assess for dysmorphic features.

How to summarise your findings

'From my examination, I have found that _____

- has difficulties with social communication, as demonstrated by their _____ (difficulty with maintaining eye contact, limited use of gesture, poor initiation of play with me and/or their parents, difficulties with imaginative role play, etc.).
- has the following physical features suggestive of a diagnosis of _____, which may be associated with this child's autism.
- This child also displayed difficulties with attention span, hyperactivity, and impulsivity, which may indicate that he/she has comorbid ADHD.'

Questions to prepare

- Who might refer a child with possible autism? What problems might someone with ASD present with?
- Do you know of any more formal methods for investigating ASD? Can you tell me about them?

- What investigations would you carry out in someone with ASD and severe learning difficulties?
- Who might be involved in the care of a child with ASD?
- How is ASD managed?

Top tips

- If you are having trouble engaging a child, it might be because they have impaired social skills or they don't want to engage with you. Use the parent to your advantage. Ask the parent to get involved in any games, reading a book, or in talking about colours/body parts/counting, etc. Observe the child's interaction. However, be aware that the child may demonstrate better social skills with a familiar adult!
- Do not spend too long trying to engage a child. You may run out of time for your examination.
- You cannot diagnose autism by examination alone. You could comment, if needed, that a thorough developmental history is also required.

Chapter 18 Taking a history from a child with cardiovascular disease

Michael T. Bowes and Caroline B. Jones

Key points to consider while taking a history

- The parent or carer is likely to be very knowledgeable about the child's congenital heart disease (CHD) – use this to your advantage.
- Be wary of the time limitation – take a *focused* history and don't miss key aspects.

Where to begin

It is worth starting with an open question such as 'When was _____'s CHD first diagnosed?' The parent will then often present a lot of the relevant information.

Questions to ask about the history of the presenting complaint

- When was the diagnosis made? What were the presenting symptoms?
- Try to get an accurate diagnosis from the parent rather than, for example, 'a hole in the heart'.
- What procedures have been undertaken – cardiac catheterisation, operations, what did this involve, how long was the intensive care and hospital stay?
- Was this a 'repair' or 'palliative' surgery? Are further operations or procedures expected?

Clinical Examination Skills in Paediatrics: For MRCPCH Candidates and Other Practitioners, First Edition. Edited by A. Mark Dalzell and Ian Sinha.
© 2020 John Wiley & Sons Ltd. Published 2020 by John Wiley & Sons Ltd.
Companion website: www.wiley.com/go/dalzell/paediatrics

Symptoms

- *Infants*: Increased work of breathing; cyanotic episodes; failure to thrive; excessive sweating.
- *Older children*: Palpitations; syncope; chest pains (only rarely cardiac in origin in children).
- What is the child's exercise capacity? Can the child keep up with other children their age? Do they tire easily?
- Feeding and growth: did the child ever need a nasogastric tube or gastrostomy? For infants, ask specifically about work of breathing during feeding and whether high calorie feeds have been required.

Past medical history

- Chromosomal or genetic diagnosis in association with CHD?
- It is worth asking relevant questions here rather than completing a full review of symptoms.
- Infections – children with CHD are particularly prone to recurrent upper and lower respiratory tract infections.
- What other professionals are involved? Dietician, speech and language therapist?
- Dental visits and caries?

Medications and vaccination history

- Current medications and medications given prior to surgical repair.
- Are they up to date with routine vaccinations, are they prescribed respiratory syncytial virus or flu vaccines in winter?

Birth history

- CHD is seen more commonly in premature and low-birth-weight infants and this may complicate surgical management.
- Be aware that an increasing proportion of CHD is diagnosed prenatally, typically following the 20 week anomaly scan.

Chapter 18

- Any suspicion at early screening? Was the nuchal translucency measurement raised?
- Note any maternal disease that may be associated with CHD, such as diabetes.
- Medications such as lithium or anticonvulsants can cause CHD in the fetus.

Developmental history

Development can be delayed as a result of cardiac failure in isolation, or may be seen in infants following a prolonged intensive care stay.

Family history

- CHD can be familial (rarely).
- Is there consanguinity?
- A detailed family history may be particularly important for patients with potentially inherited conditions such as cardiomyopathy or genetic arrhythmogenic disorders. In families with such conditions you should specifically ask about unexplained sudden death.
- Has the family seen a geneticist? Are they being screened for an inherited condition?

Social history

- How does _____'s CHD affect him/her and the family as a whole?
- Has school attendance been affected?
- Are there any special precautions or limitations (exercise participation)?
- Does the family have extra support or receive disability living allowance?
- What does the family find most difficult?
- In teenagers it may be worth asking about their understanding of their condition and discussing compliance.

How to summarise your findings

This should be succinct, aiming for two or three sentences as the examiner will be observing throughout.

Give the child's name, age, diagnosis, previous interventions, and current symptoms.

Questions to prepare

- Be able to formulate a management plan and suggest appropriate investigations.
- Be prepared to discuss psychological aspects and physical issues that might affect quality of life.
- Know the routine vaccination schedule and things that might be different for children with CHD or immune dysfunction (22q11 deletion).

Top tips

- Remember to engage the child (provide toys to play with) and ask teenagers questions directly.
- It is worth asking the parent if they have the child's red book or health record to look at the growth chart.
- 'Is there anything important you feel I've missed out' is always a good question to put to the parent or older child towards the end and may yield something important.
- Think about aspects of management planning as you go, as the examiners are likely to focus on this during the question section.

Chapter 19 **Taking a history from a child with asthma**

Sarah J. Mayell and Anna Shawcross

Key points to consider while taking a history

- Start with an open question – allow the child (or parent if the child is too young) to tell you their perception of the 'problem'/their opinion of their asthma control. This will hopefully guide you to ensure you cover the points the examiner is looking for.
- Frequency and severity of interval symptoms – do these occur several times a day, daily, weekly, or even less?
  - Wheeze, cough (may be daytime/night-time/both), chest tightness, and exercise-induced symptoms?
  - How often does the child use a bronchodilator? Does it relieve his or her symptoms?
- Establish the frequency and severity of exacerbations:
  - What is the typical pattern of exacerbations?
  - How often has this occurred in the last (for example) year?
  - What treatment has been required? For example, has the child been managed in primary care with additional steroids/hospital admission/intravenous treatments?
  - Any obvious precipitants, e.g. allergen exposure, viral upper respiratory tract infections?
  - Has the child ever needed critical care admission?

Clinical Examination Skills in Paediatrics: For MRCPCH Candidates and Other Practitioners, First Edition. Edited by A. Mark Dalzell and Ian Sinha.
© 2020 John Wiley & Sons Ltd. Published 2020 by John Wiley & Sons Ltd.
Companion website: www.wiley.com/go/dalzell/paediatrics

- How is the child's asthma affecting his or her life? How much school is missed? Is the child limited by his or her asthma, e.g. unable to participate in sport?

Medication

- What asthma treatments does the child take?
  - Clarify the strength of inhalers, e.g. beclometasone can be 50, 100, or 200 µg/puff.
  - Clarify the device used – if using an metered-dose inhaler (MDI), does the child use a spacer? What kind? Does the child have a different device, e.g. breath-actuated, for use at school?
  - Some children may use a regime where they specifically take inhaled corticosteroids as and when needed.
  - When was the child's inhaler technique last checked?
- Discuss compliance. This is absolutely vital in an asthma history.

Additional history

- Does the child have eczema/hay fever/allergies?
- Is the child exposed to environmental cigarette smoke?
- Ask about any damp, dust, building work or mould in the home, and any known exposure to air pollutants.
- Does the family have pets? Has the child had allergy testing?
- Any other ongoing medical issues?
- Does the child have an asthma nurse? How often does the nurse make contact with the child?
- Does the child have an asthma management plan to guide carers in the event of an exacerbation and do carers use it?
- Does the child receive seasonal flu immunisation?

Top tips

- If the child is on lots of asthma treatments but still very symptomatic, there are three main possibilities:
  1 The child does not actually have asthma or the child has asthma and an additional problem – be prepared to discuss differential diagnoses.

Chapter 19

2 Non-compliance – be prepared to discuss strategies to clarify and address this.

3 The child does, in fact, have uncontrolled asthma and needs additional treatment.

- Be aware of the British Thoracic Society asthma guidelines and be prepared to discuss when to 'step-up' treatment, but also when to 'step-down' treatment.

- It is useful (in real life as well as in exams!) to be aware of the different colours of inhaler devices, what drugs are contained in combination preparations, and the appearances/colours of different spacer devices.

Chapter 20 Taking a history from a child with cystic fibrosis

Antonia K.S. McBride and Kevin W. Southern

Key points to consider while taking a history

The management of cystic fibrosis (CF) is focused on giving children the best possible quality of life throughout their childhood, and maintaining good health. This is in stark contrast to CF management in years gone by, when survival to adulthood was considered an acceptable outcome. The main advances in CF have come from greater understanding and categorisation of the basic cellular defects, and the gene mutations that cause these.

The cornerstones of the management of CF are to:

1 keep the airways as healthy as possible, including efforts to both prevent and proactively treat infections
2 maintain good nutritional status
3 maintain a healthy and active lifestyle.

The therapies required to achieve these goals can be time-consuming and onerous, but are vital. It is important to remember and acknowledge the impact of these therapies on the child's social and family life, and to accept that not all children can complete all their therapies all of the time. This should be explored in your history.

Clinical Examination Skills in Paediatrics: For MRCPCH Candidates and Other Practitioners, First Edition. Edited by A. Mark Dalzell and Ian Sinha.
© 2020 John Wiley & Sons Ltd. Published 2020 by John Wiley & Sons Ltd.
Companion website: www.wiley.com/go/dalzell/paediatrics

Much of the history-taking process will be similar to that of a child with any chronic illness, but there are some important specific considerations in the history of a child with CF, as follows.

- The child is managed by a multidisciplinary team, including physicians and specialist allied health professionals. You must be able to discuss the roles that each of the members of the team plays in the management of the child's CF. You should also be aware that children are managed within regional CF networks, comprising both a local and a tertiary team. There is regional variation around how these networks work.
- Monitoring of children with CF in clinic is about spotting deteriorations over time (which could be detected during the structured annual review process that children with CF undergo), and also being alert to subtle changes in their health that may indicate a serious underlying problem (hence regular follow-up every few weeks in clinic, and close communication between the family and the CF team). To understand the child's overall health status you should ask about their annual review process and results over the last few years. Children and adolescents should live as normal a life as possible, with some extra considerations around CF. The social history is the part of the consultation when you should be asking the child two questions: 'How does CF affect your ability to lead a normal life?' and 'How do aspects of your life (e.g. school, family, hobbies, lifestyle choices) affect your ability to manage your CF?'

Background

- How was the child diagnosed? Was CF identified through newborn screening, complications in the newborn period (e.g. meconium ileus), or in later childhood?
  - Most children with CF are now identified in the newborn period. It is useful to ask about how the family felt, if their baby was identified by screening. Unlike the past, when

children with CF were picked up because they were unwell,
families of babies identified on screening will have received
the diagnosis out of the blue, and their beautiful, bouncing
baby may have had no symptoms at all.

- Genotype. Most families will know this, as it has become
increasingly relevant with the advent of new therapies that
target specific mutations.
- Family tree. Any other family members with CF? Having previous experience of a child with CF in the family is not neces-
sarily an advantage. The family may have recollections of an
unwell relative in the past, although the management and
outcomes of CF have progressed significantly in recent years.

Respiratory status

You must gauge the severity of the child's lung disease, and
establish whether there are recent changes in symptoms that
might require intervention.

- Symptoms – cough, sputum (colour and volume), wheeze,
breathlessness, nasal symptoms of discharge or blockage. Of
these, cough is a particularly good indicator of whether there may
be airway inflammation. Ask about whether the child has these
symptoms on a good day, or just when they have an infection.
- Microbiology – what organisms do they grow? Has the child
ever grown *Pseudomonas*, non-tuberculous mycobacteria, or
other significant pathogens? When was the last growth? What
eradication treatment has the child had?
- Antibiotics:
  - Are these oral or nebulised?
  - Has the child had any infective pulmonary exacerbations of
  CF requiring a change to antibiotics? Did the child need
  intravenous (IV) antibiotics, and were these given at home
  or in hospital?
  - Does the child need regular IV antibiotics, and if so do they
  have a port-a-cath?

Chapter 20

- Admissions for IV antibiotics are disruptive for the family and for the child's social life and education. A child will only be admitted if really necessary, e.g. because of a decline in symptoms necessitating IV antibiotics and only if medical, social, or logistical reasons prevent the child being given them at home.
- When were the last lung function tests (if the child is old enough), and have these changed over the years? Lung function does fluctuate, but changes in the forced expiratory volume in one second (FEV_1) of more than 10% are more likely to be significant. FEV_1 is important in CF as a decline in this parameter is associated with an increased risk of mortality. Some centres are now using the lung clearance index (LCI) to evaluate the severity of lung disease in CF.
- Ask about physiotherapy, including the techniques used, and the burden this places on the family.
- Many children now have nebulised mucolytics, such as hypertonic saline or DNAase. Ask how these are administered (there are various nebuliser kits), how frequently, how long they take, and how frequently a dose is missed.
- Ask whether the child has had allergic bronchopulmonary aspergillosis (ABPA).
- Compliance with medications/physiotherapy. Taking medications, particularly nebulisers, and undergoing physiotherapy is both time-consuming and boring. Ask how compliant the child is with these treatments, find out how the child fits them into their day, and establish whether any recent changes in family circumstances (e.g. new school or a new baby) might affect compliance.

Nutritional status

A great deal of emphasis is placed on good nutrition in CF because there is a strong correlation between nutritional status and respiratory function, and indeed mortality. Important areas to cover include the following.

- Weight gain/centile, and whether this has been of concern to the parents, child, or dietician.
- Whether the child takes pancreatic supplements (Creon), and what quantity is taken.
- Whether the child has a good appetite, and whether this gets worse during exacerbations of CF.
- Is there a need for nutritional supplements/overnight feeds? Does the child have a percutaneous gastrostomy (PEG)?
- Does the child have constipation/distal intestinal obstruction syndrome (DIOS)? If so, is any treatment needed? DIOS is a condition unique to CF, in which viscous mucus and faecal matter collect in the distal small bowel and cause symptoms of bowel obstruction. Children with CF may also be prone to constipation without progressing to DIOS. Aggressive laxative treatment is usually successful in DIOS, but occasionally surgical disimpaction is required.

Exercise and lifestyle

- Daily physical activity is one of the best forms of physiotherapy for children with CF, and also has the benefit of helping them to maintain as normal a lifestyle as possible.
- Does the child exercise every day? What do they do?
- What is the child's exercise tolerance/restriction of activity?

Number of days off school
Has there been any change in school attendance recently? Poor school attendance should lead you to clarify why this is so. With the exception of half days off to attend clinic, a child with CF would be expected to be attending school, and a recent decline in attendance may signal deteriorating health.

Effect of CF on social and family life/holidays/activities
Maintaining a normal lifestyle is important, but school trips/sleepovers/holidays can become difficult if the child requires large amounts of medication, uses a nebuliser, or requires

Chapter 20

overnight feeds. If the child's social or sporting activities have declined recently, ask why. Is the child too unwell?

Smoking (in the household, and in the child if old enough)

It goes without saying that a person with CF should be discouraged from smoking. Smoking in the family should also be discouraged, both because of the potential harms of passive smoking and in order to reduce the likelihood of the child taking up smoking when he or she becomes older.

Immunisations

Are these up to date (including influenza)?

Social/family support

The practical and emotional burden of caring for a child with CF, even when they are well, is heavy. Sharing these responsibilities with other members of the family will enable the parents to have some 'time off' – for instance, if a grandparent can perform physiotherapy, he or she can look after the child overnight without treatment being affected.

Involvement in research

Most families of a child with CF will be aware of recent research into 'transformational' treatments, which are the first drugs to target the cause of CF rather than the symptoms. Ivacaftor (Kalydeco) is a potentiator that increases cystic fibrosis transmembrane regulator (CFTR) function in patients with the G551D mutation (about 4% of patients with CF). It has been shown to improve lung function in these patients and has been licensed in the UK for use in patients over the age of six with the G551D mutation. Orkambi (a combination of ivacaftor and lumacaftor) has a less dramatic effect on lung function in patients who are homozygous for the delta F508 mutation, the most common CF mutation in the UK. You may meet a patient in the exam who is on ivacaftor.

Chapter 20

Multisystem complications of CF

- Sinopulmonary (nasal polyps/rhinosinusitis).
- CF-related diabetes.
- CF-related liver disease.
- Arthritis.
- Allergies (particularly *Aspergillus*).

Top tips

School attendance can be a sensitive marker of how well the child is and how well the family is coping with the child's CF. A decline in attendance should be a prompt to ask what else has changed recently and what, exactly, is stopping the child from going to school.

Unlike other chronic illnesses, children with CF are strongly discouraged from being in contact with each other because of cross-infection risks. Ask the family if they use social media, internet forums, or apps to keep up with CF news and to contact other families.

If the child is old enough, ask how the process of transition to adult services is going. What stage has the child reached in the transition process? How does the child feel about it? Does the child have any concerns?

Chapter 21 **Taking a history from a child with inflammatory bowel disease (Crohn disease and ulcerative colitis)**

Anastasia Konidari and A. Mark Dalzell

Key points to consider while taking a history

- Any persistent disturbance in bowel habit from the norm requires evaluation, particularly when associated with a change in demeanour.
- Loose and/or frequent stools may be a sign of intestinal malabsorption (coeliac disease being the most common cause) or a sign of colitis due to Crohn disease or ulcerative colitis.
- Loose stool with soiling is most likely to be due to mega-rectum and overflow diarrhoea.
- Rectal bleeding is a cardinal feature of inflammatory bowel disease and requires endoscopic evaluation.
- If rectal bleeding is painful, consider constipation, anal fissure, or perianal Crohn disease.
- If rectal bleeding is intermittent in an otherwise well child consider rectal polyp or threadworm infestation.
- Ulcerative colitis is most likely with a history of loose stools of recent onset with overt or intermittent rectal bleeding, particularly if there is urgency to pass stool and a need to get out of bed to go to the toilet.

Clinical Examination Skills in Paediatrics: For MRCPCH Candidates and Other Practitioners, First Edition. Edited by A. Mark Dalzell and Ian Sinha.
© 2020 John Wiley & Sons Ltd. Published 2020 by John Wiley & Sons Ltd.
Companion website: www.wiley.com/go/dalzell/paediatrics

- Crohn disease is most likely with a history of change in bowel habit with abdominal pain as a feature – usually of a few months' standing.
- Inflammatory bowel disease should be a consideration in any child with growth failure, particularly if abdominal pain and change of bowel habit are evident.
- Essential elements in the history of a child with suspected inflammatory bowel disease:
  - duration, type, and location of abdominal pain
  - lower abdominal pain is indicative of hind-gut or colonic inflammation.
- Peri-umbilical abdominal pain is indicative of mid-gut disturbance:
  - assess the change in bowel habit and type of rectal bleeding.
- Loss of appetite, reduction in level of activity, school absence, and loss of weight are of significance:
  - is there a family history of Inflammatory bowel disease?

Questions to prepare

- How do you investigate a child with suspected inflammatory bowel disease?
- How do you manage a child with Crohn disease?
- How do you manage a patient with ulcerative colitis?
- Distinguish inflammatory bowel disease from recurrent abdominal pain syndrome.

Top tips

- Does the child seem unwell?
- 'Unprovoked fatigue means disease' – *Hippocratic Writings*, Aphorisms, Section II, 5, p. 209 (ed. GER Lloyd; Penguin, London).
- Summarising the features of abdominal pain and bowel disturbance will point to a diagnosis.
- Evaluate growth and growth charts.

- 'Surgical causes' of rectal bleeding are associated with an 'acute abdomen'.
- Volvulus, intussusception, and peptic ulceration may present with rectal bleeding but also with severe acute abdominal pain and often vomiting.
- Congenital polyposis syndromes such as Peutz–Jeghers syndrome and familial polyposis coli are less frequent causes of rectal bleeding in childhood.
- 'Do not judge the stools by their quantity but by their quality and the manner of them, what is needful and comfortable for the patient' – *Hippocratic Writings*, Aphorisms, Section I, 23, p. 209 (ed. GER Lloyd; Penguin, London).
- Inflammatory markers (erythrocyte sedimentation rate [ESR], C-reactive protein [CRP], platelets) – if not raised do not exclude inflammatory bowel disease.

Chapter 22 Taking a history from a child with renal transplant

Dean Wallace

Key points to consider while taking a history

Try to categorise the history into pre-, peri-, and post-transplant sections. This will allow you to work logically through questions and organise the presentation of your findings.

Pre-transplant
- What is the child's underlying diagnosis and how old were they at diagnosis?
- What were the symptoms leading to diagnosis?
- The length between diagnosis and transplant may give you an indication of the rate of renal decline – this may be worth commenting on.
- What were the complications or consequences of their chronic renal impairment? Anaemia? Mineral bone disease? Failure to thrive? Short stature?
- The impact of the disease may be things like fatigue/malaise/inability to participate in sports or activities, previous fractures, recurrent infections, multiple clinic attendances/admissions, missed exams, repeated school years, etc.

Dialysis
- The majority of patients will have been dialysed for some period of time before transplant.

Clinical Examination Skills in Paediatrics: For MRCPCH Candidates and Other Practitioners, First Edition. Edited by A. Mark Dalzell and Ian Sinha.
© 2020 John Wiley & Sons Ltd. Published 2020 by John Wiley & Sons Ltd.
Companion website: www.wiley.com/go/dalzell/paediatrics

- Pre-emptive transplants are now increasing in numbers where organ availability is sufficient for patients who are not yet in end-stage renal failure.
- Ask about which type of dialysis the child was on – peritoneal or haemodialysis (via a Hickman line/arteriovenous fistula) and for how long.
- Ask about any specific complications associated with dialysis, i.e. haemo-line thrombus/migration/infection/revision/peritonitis/peritoneal dialysis catheter revision (omentectomy), etc.

Peri-transplant

- Identify if the transplant was from a deceased donor (DDKT) or a live-related donor (LRDKT) or the rarer altruistic living donors.
- The family or child may even know the degree of mismatch or if the transplant was blood group incompatible – so it's worth asking! Mismatch is expressed as three digits, with 0-0-0 being human leukocyte antigen (HLA) identical and ranging to 1-0-1, 1-1-0, etc. The family or child may disclose that it was ABO incompatible.
- Ask if the graft functioned immediately with urine production and a fall in creatinine. DDKTs more commonly exhibit delayed graft function and acute tubular necrosis (ATN), which is related to the ischaemic out-of-body time. The child may have required a short period of dialysis post transplant.
- Ask about any complications and length of stay.

Post transplant

- This is really about how the child is doing now.
- Ask about current renal function. The child or parent will usually know the baseline creatinine.
- Ask if any biopsies have been required and what they demonstrated, i.e. rejection, calcineurin inhibitor toxicity (tacrolimus/ciclosporin), etc.
- Ask about any confirmed and treated episodes of rejection.
- Ask about immunosuppression. Most are on one or a combination of the drugs tacrolimus (Prograf/Modigraf/Advagraf/

Adoport), mycophenolate mofetil (CellCept/Myfortic), aza-thioprine, sirolimus, and prednisolone.

- Many transplant centres have now adapted a drug protocol that advocates the early withdrawal of steroids, but ask about the effects of long-term steroid use.

Functional impact

- The examiners are looking for candidates who collect, organise, and present the right information but also who understand the functional impact of the process on the child, the family, and wider society.
- Make a point of presenting the issues of lost school days, missed exams, reduced participation in sports/team activities, repeated school years, inability to take holidays, psychosocial effects of chronic steroid use, fear of graft rejection, uncertain future, lifelong immunosuppression, and the societal and familial cost of chronic disease.

How to summarise your findings

'I would like to present the case history of Jack, who is a 7-year-old boy who has undergone a renal transplant.

Jack was a term delivery, 3.5 kg with a non-significant antenatal and perinatal history. Apart from the issues pertaining to his transplant, which I will explore shortly, he has no other significant medical conditions and has no known drug allergies. His immunisation schedule is up to date and he is neuro-developmentally appropriate for his age. He is one of three children. His mother is X years old and a housewife and his father is Y years old and a builder. He is currently in year X at St John's primary school.

Jack presented at the age of 4 years with a nephrotic syndrome which was unresponsive to a month of oral corticosteroids and three doses of intravenous methylprednisolone. A renal biopsy demonstrated advanced focal sclerosing glomerulosclerosis (FSGS) and he was trialled on several immunosuppressants, such as ciclosporin, which failed to keep him in remission. His renal function rapidly declined and a pre-emptive LRDKT from his mother was undertaken in December of last year. His mother tells me that the mismatch was 1-0-1 and they were blood-group compatible. There was no period of dialysis before the transplant.

Jack's mother tells me that the graft functioned immediately and his serum creatinine fell sharply to his baseline in the 30s. He was an in-patient for 14 days and was discharged to outpatient follow-up. His immunosuppressant regime now consists of tacrolimus 2 mg bd and mycophenolate mofetil (MMF) 500 mg bd.

He has required two post-transplant renal biopsies, each because of sudden rises in his creatinine. Neither has shown rejection, only tacrolimus toxicity due to high serum levels. He must drink an oral fluid target of 1.5–2 litres/day and his blood pressure is well controlled on no antihypertensives. Clinic visits have demonstrated a normal protein level in the urine. His family are aware that FSGS can recur in the transplant graft.

Jack is now attending the transplant clinic on a 2-monthly basis depending on his blood and urine results.

On specific questioning about the functional impact of his transplant Jack mentions that his life is easier now and that he has to take fewer medications. His mother discussed the many previous admissions with oedema and proteinuria and the long-term effects of corticosteroids, namely behavioural and facial changes in Jack. His mother mentioned the spectre of disease recurrence in the graft, but that Jack's current situation is far better than his pre-transplant situation and multiple hospital admissions. Jack is settling well back at school with the support of his teachers, school nurse, and transplant nurse specialist.'

Chapter 23 **Taking a history from a child with diabetes**

Mark Deakin

Background

The prevalence of childhood diabetes is increasing and currently stands at 100–140 per 100 000 children. There are approximately 23 000 children with diabetes in the UK: 97% have type 1 diabetes, the remaining 3% have type 2/maturity-onset diabetes of the young (MODY). Very rarely a child will develop diabetes as a result of another medical condition, such as cystic fibrosis-related diabetes or after administration of high-dose steroids – in the treatment of cancer or systemic disease.

Children with diabetes may present to hospital with hypo- or hyperglycaemia or with another medical complaint that will directly affect their diabetes such as an infection.

Diabetes in children may not demonstrate the classic long-term sequelae noted in adults but a careful history and thorough examination will reveal those at risk.

How has the child been recently?

- Has the child had any episodes of diabetic keto-acidosis (DKA)?
- When was the child last seen in the diabetes clinic – does the child or parent remember what the last HbA1c measurement was?

Clinical Examination Skills in Paediatrics: For MRCPCH Candidates and Other Practitioners, First Edition. Edited by A. Mark Dalzell and Ian Sinha.
© 2020 John Wiley & Sons Ltd. Published 2020 by John Wiley & Sons Ltd.
Companion website: www.wiley.com/go/dalzell/paediatrics

How did the child present initially?

- When was the child diagnosed with diabetes?
- Was the diagnosis recent (within the last six months)?
- What has been happening with the child's blood glucose readings?
- Has the child come to the end of the honeymoon period during which they stop making endogenous insulin?
- High or low blood glucose?
- Vomiting/nausea/abdominal pain?
- Deep sighing (Kussmaul) breathing?
- Sepsis?

Has the child had symptoms of hypo- or hyperglycaemia?

Symptoms of hypoglycaemia	Symptoms of hyperglycaemia
• Becoming sweaty • Poor concentration • Becoming hungry • Becoming angry or argumentative • Having mild abdominal pain • Shaking (or feeling wobbly) • Having glazed eyes • Pallor	• Polydipsia • Polyuria • Lethargy • Weight loss • Secondary enuresis • Poor concentration • Hunger • Deep sighing breathing

Past medical history

- Does the child have any comorbidities?
  - Thyroid deficiency/coeliac disease/Addison disease?
  - Pernicious anaemia/rheumatoid arthritis?

- When was the child diagnosed with diabetes? How has their control been?
- Have there been any recent periods of illness?
- Any previous DKA?
- Any critical care admissions?
- Low mood/depression/previous self-harm (physical or with medication)?
- Does the child regularly see a dentist? High blood glucose causes glucose to be high in other bodily fluids, increasing the risk of infections and tooth decay (also remember that hypoglycaemia is treated with sugary drinks/snacks).

Medicines/immunisations/allergy

- What type of insulin(s)?
- What are the injection times?
- Who does the injections (at home/school)?
- How many units?
- Have there been any missed doses?
- Has there been any equipment failure (pens/pump/blood glucose meter)?
- Is the child up to date with his or her immunisations? Children with diabetes should be offered the seasonal influenza vaccination by their GP.
- Is the child taking any other medication, e.g. thyroxine (thyroid disease) or hydrocortisone/fludrocortisone (Addison disease).

You may see different insulin regimens in use. The most common is 'basal bolus' as this gives the most practical physiological control. Pre-mixed twice daily injections avoid the need to inject at school – some families find that this is best for them. Insulin pump therapy is becoming more common as it gives much more refined glucose control. However, it does require carbohydrate counting and more frequent blood glucose testing, especially before food is eaten.

Chapter 23

- Basal/bolus (or multiple daily injections [MDIs]) with approximately 50% long-acting (Lantus [insulin glargine] or Levemir [insulin detemir]) at bedtime and 50% in divided doses with meals – the child may take variable amounts if they carbohydrate count and use an insulin-to-carbohydrate ratio.
- Twice daily pre-mixed (30% short acting/70% long acting) – two-thirds in the morning and one-third in the evening.
- Continuous subcutaneous insulin infusion (CSII or insulin pump). This gives a continuous background infusion of short-acting insulin with bolus doses based on carbohydrate in the child's meals.

Family history

- Is there a family history of diabetes/autoimmune disease?
- Type 1 diabetes is more common if there is a family history (3% likelihood if the mother has type 1 diabetes, 7% likelihood if the father has type 1 diabetes, 30% likelihood if both parents have type 1 diabetes, 10% likelihood if a sibling has type 1 diabetes (Delli et al. 2010).

Social history

- Who lives at home?
- Who does the injections at home/school?
- Do the parents live together? If not, does the child spend time in different locations during the week/weekend?
- What year is the child in at school?
- What are the child's career intentions?
- Is there any involvement with social services?
- Does the family receive Disability Living Allowance?

Diabetes has a major psychosocial impact on both the affected child and his or her parents. Apart from the medical management of the condition there is the change in social dynamic at school and the impact that this has on peer relationships. Children with diabetes receive more input from teachers, especially at primary school if they need help performing blood glucose testing or injections. They may be seen as different because they are allowed to eat first or at times when their classmates are not, such as before PE.

Diabetes can restrict access to certain jobs, especially those that involve transportation and the armed forces. Any child with diabetes who applies for a driving licence will have to complete an additional medical questionnaire and, when approved, will receive a shortened driving licence (between one and three years' duration); this is renewed each time depending on their glycaemic control and perceived risk to other road users – people with diabetes do not need to retake their driving test each time the licence is renewed.

Reference

Delli, A.J., Larsson, H.E., Ivarsson, S.-A. et al. (2010). Type 1 diabetes. In: *Textbook of Diabetes*, 4e (eds. R.I.G. Holt, C.S. Cockram, A. Flyvbjerg, et al.). Oxford: Wiley-Blackwell.

Chapter 23

Chapter 24 Taking a history from a child with a rheumatological condition

Gavin Cleary

Background

- Musculoskeletal symptoms are a common reason for referral by GPs to paediatric services. Musculoskeletal pain and stiffness in particular are frequent presenting features and candidates should be able to elicit details relating to onset, site, severity, impact on function, and any associated non-articular symptoms.
- There are (broad) differential diagnoses (ranging in severity) for common symptoms such as joint pain or limping and key features in a history should guide the candidate to the correct diagnosis or at least a working differential diagnosis.
- Candidates must have a knowledge of normal development of gait and also be aware of changes in normal joint range of movement at different ages.
- Musculoskeletal symptoms may be associated with multisystem diseases such as juvenile dermatomyositis (JDM), juvenile systemic lupus erythematosus (jSLE), or systemic vasculitides such as Henoch–Schönlein purpura (HSP) and Kawasaki disease. A history may therefore be focused on, for example, joint symptoms but must include a review of systems, relevant family history, medication, and, where relevant, a psychosocial history.

Clinical Examination Skills in Paediatrics: For MRCPCH Candidates and Other Practitioners, First Edition. Edited by A. Mark Dalzell and Ian Sinha.
© 2020 John Wiley & Sons Ltd. Published 2020 by John Wiley & Sons Ltd.
Companion website: www.wiley.com/go/dalzell/paediatrics

Children with chronic inflammatory disease such as juvenile idiopathic arthritis (JIA) are managed by multidisciplinary teams and may now access a very wide range of immunomodulatory drugs, including biological therapies.

- Candidates may be asked to elicit specific histories relating to the management of rheumatological conditions.
- Candidates must have a working knowledge of a team approach to chronic rheumatological disease.

Where to begin

- Always engage both the child (age appropriate) and parent/carer in the history.
- Remember that children may find it difficult to articulate symptoms such as pain and stiffness so try to find appropriate language, e.g. 'hurts' or 'hard to move', or interpret language the child may use by collaboration with the parent.
- Remember that some articular symptoms may be referred from other sites, e.g. pain in the knee referred from pathology in the hip

Essential components to the musculoskeletal history

- Joint pain/arthralgia
  - Location and characteristics
    - Severity, precipitating and relieving factors, radiation, and diurnal variation.
  - Onset – acute or chronic? This will help distinguish cause.
  - Exacerbation by *rest* ('gelling') – for example symptoms may be more pronounced early in the morning after rising from bed, and improve with activity. This suggests an inflammatory process – is there an associated history of joint swelling?
  - Exacerbation by *activity* suggests a biomechanical process – investigate sporting or other physical activities and association with joint hypermobility.

Chapter 24

- Associated non-articular symptoms, including fever, weight loss, fatigue, and rashes, must be sought.
- Muscle pain and weakness
  - Inflammatory muscle disease (usually JDM, but may occur in 'overlap' with another autoimmune disease, e.g. jSLE) associated with skin features such as heliotrope rash and Gottron's papules.
- Elicit functional difficulties and the impact of symptoms on activities of daily living such as schooling.

Remember to seek non-articular symptoms – *always consider as alerts ('red flags') to possible serious pathology:*

- fever
- night sweats
- night pain
- weight loss
- pallor or bruising
- abdominal pain
- malaise/lethargy
- weakness
- rash
- disability associated with symptoms.

Diagnostic categories for musculoskeletal symptoms may include any of the following, and this surgical sieve approach is recommended when candidates approach history-taking at this station:

- congenital
- normal variant
- inflammatory
- orthopaedic/mechanical
- neoplastic
- infective
- metabolic
- traumatic

- haematological
- iatrogenic
- chronic non-inflammatory pain syndromes.

Common conditions

1 Inflammatory disease
   - JIA – defined by *onset* pattern (first six months of disease) of *persistent* arthritis:
     - Oligoarthritis – fewer than four joints. If additional joints become involved after six months the classification becomes *extended oligoarthritis*.
     - Polyarthritis – five or more joints involved in the first six months of disease.
     - Systemic arthritis – associated with quotidian fever, rash, serositis, hepatosplenomegaly, and lymphadenopathy
     - Psoriatic arthritis – remember to seek a family history of psoriasis.
     - Enthesitis-related arthritis – associated with human leukocyte antigen (HLA) B27 status.
   - *Key point*: all JIA sub-types may be associated with uveitis – all children with a rheumatological condition should be screened by an ophthalmologist.
2 Non inflammatory disease
   - Hypermobility syndromes:
     - Commonly associated with biomechanical pattern musculoskeletal pain.
     - Ehlers–Danlos syndrome – look for associated symptoms such as skin laxity, easy bruising, and hypertrophic scarring.
     - Marfan syndrome – enquire for associated scoliosis and anterior chest wall deformities. Children should have cardiac surveillance.
     - *Key point*: infants and younger children will often have hypermobile joints – history of associated features to distinguish normal variation from pathological hypermobility.

Chapter 24

- Chronic amplified musculoskeletal pain syndromes:
  - May be associated with hypermobility.
  - Pain often disproportionate to initiating trigger, with allodynia (hyperalgesia).
  - May be associated autonomic dysfunction – enquire regarding peripheral blood flow changes and abnormal sudomotor activity.
  - May be associated psychosocial distress factors.
- Apophysitis of tibial tuberosity – Osgood–Schlatter disease.
- Specific hip disorders including Perthes disease and slipped upper femoral epiphysis (SUFE).

3 Autoimmune inflammatory syndromes
- jSLE
  - Photosensitive malar rash.
  - Malaise and lethargy common at presentation.
  - Any organ system can be involved – detailed full review of systems is mandatory.
- JDM
  - Inflammatory pattern muscle pain and weakness.
  - Primarily proximal muscle groups affected, e.g. difficulty standing from sitting.
  - Associated skin lesions are typically heliotrope discoloration of upper eyelids and Gottron's papules on the extensor aspects of the small joints of the hands. May be vasculitis lesions elsewhere.
- Juvenile scleroderma
  - Classified as localised (linear scleroderma and morphoea) or systemic sclerosis.
  - Localised disease often has subtle symptoms such as itchiness of the affected area. May have significant cosmetic adverse effects, especially if it involves the head and neck.
  - Systemic sclerosis may involve internal organs, requiring detailed system review.

- Systemic vasculitis syndromes
  - Very variable phenotypes, commonest HSP and Kawasaki disease.
  - Multisystem disorders are usually associated with systemic inflammatory responses and fever that cannot be explained by an infective cause.

Screening history

Candidates should be familiar with the screening tool paediatric Gait Arms Legs Spine (pGALS) (available at https://www.versusarthritis.org).

The following key questions taken from pGALS should help alert candidates to significant musculoskeletal problems, which can then be explored in more detail:

1 Do you have any pain or difficulty in moving your arms, legs, neck, or back?
2 When you get dressed, are you able to do this yourself without any help?
3 Can you walk up and down the stairs without any problems?

Management of rheumatological conditions

All chronic inflammatory disease is managed holistically by a multidisciplinary team approach. Candidates should be aware of broad principles as follows:

- Medical therapies to suppress inflammation (immunosuppressant therapy). May be delivered locally, e.g. intra-articular steroid injection in JIA, or systemically, including disease-modifying anti-rheumatic agents such as methotrexate and, increasingly, use of biological agents such as anti-cytokine therapies. There may be associated risk of adverse events such as sepsis.
- Oral corticosteroid use may be associated with significant toxicity and candidates should be aware of these features.

Chapter 24

- Physical therapy is required to restore and maintain musculoskeletal function.
- Nursing support regarding disease education and drug monitoring.
- Consideration of psychosocial factors, e.g. distress associated with medical therapies and procedures.
- Impact on family, including siblings, of chronic disease.

Index

Page locators in **bold** indicate tables. This index uses letter-by-letter alphabetization.

Clinical Examination Skills in Paediatrics: For MRCPCH Candidates and Other Practitioners, First Edition. Edited by A. Mark Dalzell and Ian Sinha.
© 2020 John Wiley & Sons Ltd. Published 2020 by John Wiley & Sons Ltd.
Companion website: www.wiley.com/go/dalzell/paediatrics